Code: Red, White, and Blue

CODE: RED, WHITE, and BLUE

A Revolutionary Solution to Saving America's Healthcare System

Shary Connella

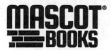

www.mascotbooks.com

Code: Red, White, and Blue

For more information, please contact:
Mascot Books
620 Herndon Parkway #320
Herndon, VA 20170
info@mascotbooks.com

CPSIA Code: PBANG0918A
Library of Congress Control Number: 2018909532
ISBN-13: 978-1-64307-226-5

Printed in the United States

This book is dedicated to my mother, Mary Etta Philpot Connella. Although you left our earth, I hear your wings flap as you soar without pain. I hear you whisper your wisdom in my ears still to this day. May your legacy live for generations to come in this book.

This book is also dedicated to my father, Earl Thomas Connella Jr., whose strength, intelligence, courage, and moral compass guide me every day to stand up for our rights.

And lastly, I dedicate this book to everyone who has touched my heart; you are the most valued treasures in my life.

Contents

Foreword

"*Code: Red, White, and Blue's* healthcare
solution puts people before profiteering."

Marianne Williamson

#1 *New York Times* bestselling author, lecturer, activist,
and internationally acclaimed spiritual teacher

Preface

About two decades ago, I began a career in *healthcare* after years working as a photojournalist and creative photographer. Over the past twenty years, I've watched our *healthcare* system decline firsthand. The free fall has hurt patients, created distrust in my industry, and is now paralyzing Washington, where our elected officials simply cannot get it right.

I was finally driven to pen my own manuscript as an act of public service, a call for us all to take control not only of our own health but also our nation's *healthcare* programs. We, collectively, have a strong role to play in changing our nation's health culture and trajectory. This moment in history is a real crisis—and the stagnation is killing people, good people, every day.

In *Code: Red, White, and Blue*, I share personal stories and insights from my career, and I offer real solutions on how to fix our problems.

In hospitals, the phrase *code: blue* signals an all-hands-on-deck emergency, a frantic call for doctors and nurses—often part of a select team that includes others as well—to stop what they are doing and try to save someone's life.

I am calling for a *code: red, white, and blue*—for our country.

Yes, it's a single-payer model, but one that is fair: we all contribute the same, a very American idea. A simple one too. It removes the greed and the confusion and solves a problem as we reverse years of anger and mistrust leveled at our *healthcare* system and the pharmaceutical and insurance industries as well as doctors who are caught in a conundrum that no longer allows them to heal.

I caution readers *not* to get caught up in the illusion of Democrats versus Republicans. Both parties are in bed with private insurance companies.

And if you are currently participating in Medicare or Medicaid, you are agreeing to two forms of socialized medicine.

This book came to me from participating in the Sister Giant conference in 2017 and ACIM lectures in New York City.

My goal in writing this book is to illustrate that a single-payer system is truly possible and can work in the United States.

The single-payer system will also afford physicians and healthcare practitioners the time they need to give quality care.

I hope you find *Code: Red, White and Blue* inspiring and hopeful.

Chapter 1

A Mother's Wisdom Lives On

This year marks the seventeenth anniversary of my mother's death.

Although much time has passed, I can see it so clearly, as if it is happening now.

I remember walking into my mother's hospital room on the fifth floor of Shands Teaching Hospital in Gainesville, Florida. In 1996, Gainesville was known as the home of the Fighting Gators national football champions, and my mom was no different. Mom was fighting in what was her last season on earth.

Bette Midler's song "The Rose" played on the radio as my mom sang along.

Each note gave her the courage and strength to take another breath. I recall the smell of eucalyptus oil in the air—a request by my mom to have in her room.

There was something full circle about this space and this moment. This hospital was part of the same hospital integrated delivery network less than two miles away, where she had given birth to my younger brother, Tommy, fifty-three years earlier.

Now my mother was here again. This time, in bed, all curled in a fetal position and on her side—as my dad would say, "like a baby bird, looking like a chickadee in her makeshift nest." Motionless, she would mutter a few sounds or moan as she tried to turn over on her own.

There was no pretending here. Surrounded by a medical team of three attending physicians, two fellows, six residents, and three nurses rounding, along with several family members, I felt hopeless. I knew in my heart there was nothing anyone could do. We needed a miracle, and quickly.

A miracle, at least for me, would not be defined by math or science or anything on earth at that point. I was looking for one elsewhere.

Everyone was raw with emotion and yet speechless as we all scratched our heads, uncertain of what to do or how to fix this. I wanted to cry. I did not know what to say. My voice was paralyzed with what was going on around me in her room. Time was still, yet we all knew that day was drawing closer. I wanted to grab my camera, but it wasn't appropriate because my mom was no longer recognizable.

In her day, she had given Elizabeth Taylor a run for her money as an American beauty, but that day, near her end, she looked more like a cross between a burn victim and Mr. Toad on a wild adventure to heaven. The only things keeping me from crying when I looked at Mom were her stories of attending college in the fall of 1954 at Florida State University, in Tallahassee, Florida, before she came home with appendicitis. She had met Buddy "Burt" Reynolds, a Seminoles halfback and Hollywood star who had the hots for my mom and had tried relentlessly asking her out for a date. Fate had it that she would never return to FSU to finish her degree or say yes to that date with Mr. Burt.

My dad had won her heart shortly after the soon-to-be movie star's early and unsuccessful pursuit.

Back in my mom's hospital room, across from me, was my dad, sitting by himself with his head buried in his lap—his body language said it all without saying a word.

This was very much out of his character. For most of my life, his voice overshadowed mine and my siblings, and now we found him speechless—and gutted. You could feel the palpable energy in the room. Death was nearing. Did I dare try to start conversation, engage him in idol chitchat while he tried to pick his heart off the polished floor that reflected his weary and unshaven face?

We were raised to believe that children were to be seen and not heard. And in this moment, although we were all living on our own and well over thirty years of age, this felt like no exception.

Dad had kept a family secret with God. He had been raised Catholic and had served as an altar boy until college. But here, he was putting all his faith in the doctors since he felt God had let him down when he was a young boy and would not tell us why.

I had been a photojournalist for much of my professional life. And in this hour, I was comforted by the thought of capturing these final moments on film. It was my comfort zone. And I thought I could satisfy my ADD and nerves by playing with the strap. I had been doing this dance with my camera since I was four years old. My camera was my voice and friend. I shared my truth through the lens of my camera. However, my lens was blurred in this room.

I was now hearing my mom's voice inside my head, saying she was like Humpty-Dumpty: "Humpty-Dumpty sat on a wall. / Humpty-Dumpty had a great fall; / All the King's horses and all the King's men / Couldn't put Humpty-Dumpty together again." I had reverted to nursery rhymes—a safe place, a child's place, where things were fantasy, and nothing went wrong.

Watching someone die, knowing I could not fix it or stop it, felt indescribable. I was powerless.

Today, nearly two decades later, I find myself working in the healthcare industry as an account executive for a negative-pressure-medical-device company, healing wounds. At the time of my mother's death, I worked at a company that helped women with high-risk pregnancies. In essence, my job now entails giving patients a voice in their care.

Ironically, during my mom's official diagnosis, in my own work, I represented the voices of fetuses inside their mother's wombs. The job, strangely enough, allowed me to be the liaison between physicians and patients in order to create better outcomes, saving lives while helping preserve women's dreams of becoming mothers.

Yet there I was—in a hospital, losing mine. And at the time, I could not help, could not intervene—nothing. I knew she was on her way home. Home to our Father, God.

My mother could sense what I was thinking. Mom would quietly tell me to stop worrying about her and to start meditating on living my life fully so she could stop worrying about me and keep focusing on healing. "Worry is the opposite of faith," she said.

I remember her saying, "If you can worry, you already know how to meditate." She added that instead of focusing on my problems, I should focus on the promises of God.

I did not want to focus or meditate on God. If I did that, I would have to accept defeat, at least on this plane. When she whispered those words to me again, I knew she was asking me to accept that she was going home. While sitting by her bedside, holding her hand and looking into her eyes, I could see she knew her days were numbered. I was starting to observe that, as hard as it was for all of us to see her go, it was also difficult for her to leave us as well.

My oldest sister, Tammy, and I were shaking our heads. We knew my mom's disease, called mycosis fungoides cutaneous T-cell lymphoma, had no cure. It was also wearing our mom and us all down. It was way bigger than us.

Mycosis fungoides. My mother lovingly nicknamed her disease "Motherfucker." Motherfucker because it itched like hell. She called it worse than Chinese torture. She would often say she wouldn't wish it on her worst enemy.

My mother's disease had not, however, been first diagnosed by doctors. Rather, Tammy and her husband had figured it out long before any doctor could.

One-night years before, after Tammy had settled her kids into bed, she and my brother-in-law, Dale, along with the help of his father, had decided to venture down into their basement. This was where Tammy had stored our mom's medical files from over five and half years—twenty-one doctors.

Within minutes of turning on her computer, she and Dale had begun surfing the internet, looking at thousands of pictures with symptoms similar to our mom's. With each page click, they had been piecing together our mother's medical mystery. That's how they had found it—a long name, but nearly all of her awful symptoms were in alignment with mycosis fungoides cutaneous T-cell lymphoma.

Her heart had broken at this point because we would all soon realize that our mom had been misdiagnosed. Many doctors would rubber-stamp Mom's medical files saying she did not have cancer. All she had was atopic dermatitis, which simply meant inflammation of the skin.

We would learn that her disease was very rare, and it was more common in men than in women. The chance of my mom—or any other woman, for that matter—attracting this disease was so off the charts that the doctors would tell us the odds of her having it were one in a million.

I had always known my mother was one in a million, but not this way—not with this condition.

We would learn more. Men who were diagnosed with this disease had been soldiers in the Gulf War. The cause for these men was thought to be associated with the chemical weapons they used.

But these details, as fascinating as they would become, could do little to make up for the fact that modern medicine had left my mom behind. When you're at a computer diagnosing your mother's illness after twenty-one doctors, you know that perhaps her best interests have not been served.

And now, looking back—and looking at my current career working in medicine (we'll get to how I got here later)—we can all see why relying on a vast medical system failed us.

It failed my mom.

It is failing you.

But what can you do?

Chapter 2

I Come to This Debate Honestly

Medicine and healthcare are a part of my DNA. But even as I had relatives who were physicians, I was raised in a family where thoughtful mind-body-spirit practices were decades ahead of the curve. Much of my thinking came from my mom, who was an independent spirit and who raised me with the same worldview.

On April 3, 1961, about three and a half months after John F. Kennedy was sworn in as our country's thirty-fifth president, my mother, Mary Etta Philpot Connella, labored in Cabrini Hospital, surrounded by nuns and nurses in my father's hometown of Alexandria, Louisiana. She was working hard most of the afternoon to bring a new spirit into the world—me.

At this point, I was two weeks overdue. With sweat pouring down Mom's rose-colored cheeks, below her starlight-hazel eyes, she was pushing as the nuns stood by praying.

No epidurals were on board here. In the early sixties, epidurals were being used sporadically for labor but would not gain true momentum until the seventies. So Mom, with the help of God, was doing it all on her own, inhaling and exhaling as her contractions became more and more intense.

Mom was a tiny but tough lady. Her petite body stood five feet four inches, and she weighed 125 pounds, even after ten months of being pregnant with me.

I guess it must have been pretty cozy inside her womb because my mom had been pushing to get me out most of the day.

Back then doctors did not use ultrasound to determine the sex of a baby. It was all left to fate. My dad (Earl Thomas Jr., known to most as "Tom") was outside her hospital room, hoping for a boy—a boy he could name after himself and my soon-to-become paternal grandfather.

Dad was also having fantasies of taking his son to the woods and bayous. Hunting and fishing were my dad's favorite pastimes. They were also ways he provided food for his family.

My dad was and remains very handsome. In his younger days, his head was covered in coal-black hair, with a few splashes of sleek gray. He stood six feet three inches tall, with a lean and muscular wiry-framed body. Some folks said he looked, in his early years, like the actor Robert Conrad. Conrad was best known for his role in the television series *The Wild Wild West*.

Back inside labor and delivery (L&D), I was making my entrance. At 4:34 p.m. CDT, I arrived with thick, sandy-blond, curly hair and hazel eyes—just like my mother, I was a southern belle in my own right. Sister Anna announced in her soft, gentle voice: "Your little angel is here. I think she is your smallest baby yet."

I was Mary Etta's third child and daughter, and she and my father named me Mary Sharon. But mom never wanted to call me Mary or Sharon or Mary Sharon. She wanted to call me Shary after Shari Lewis.

Lewis was an American ventriloquist, puppeteer, children's entertainer, and television-show host. She was best known as the original puppeteer of sock puppet Lamb Chop. My mom adored her but didn't like the spelling of her name, ending in *i*, and how it looked with our family's last name. So Mom dropped the *i* and added the *y*, creating *Shary*, a derivative of *Sharon*.

Even though everyone in our extended family knew how desperately my dad wanted a son, he gracefully welcomed me, his new baby girl, into the world by holding me tightly in his loving arms next to my mom's hospital bed.

He and my mother chose the name Mary for me, in honor of his mother and my mother. Nothing like a little pressure— being named after two of the most important women in my father's life.

After a few days of rest in the hospital, the three of us— Mom, Dad, and me—headed home to join my sisters, Tammy, who was three and a half, and Melody, who was two and a half.

We all lived in a small two-bedroom home off of Rutland Road, down the street from Dad's older sister, Mary Lee. Dad worked on a crew splicing cable along the road for Southern Bell. He climbed telephone poles over four hundred feet high. My mom took on the role of housewife and mother. By now, she had given up on her college education and finishing her degrees to become an architect.

In her mind, and with the expectations of that era of southern culture, it was her duty to serve my dad as his wife and to be the mother of their children. Somehow, living our dreams became more important than her following hers. She embraced motherhood and keeping our family together.

Although my father was raised Catholic and Mom Methodist, my sisters and I were not baptized in either church as newborn babies. Perhaps this was due to stories my sisters and I would hear while growing up about our parents feeling like organized religion had misused the Bible and manipulated God's word to control the masses.

Our parents believed we each had a connection with God before birth without having to go to church. A family maxim was the Golden Rule, found in the New Testament in Luke 6:31: "Do to others as you would have them do to you." It is something I try to live by today.

After I turned one, my dad was on the road with his work more than he was home. Mom was home alone with us three girls. As Dad puts it, I was "the straw that broke the camel's back." We three little girls were too much for my mom to handle alone. She asked Dad to move back to Florida, where she could be closer to her family, so they could help her raise "the girls."

Mom's hometown was Bell, Florida, not far from the Gulf of Mexico, about two and a half hours north of Tampa and forty-five minutes from Gainesville. She was missing her relatives and Florida's sunshine as well as living near a college town. The rainy, overcast days and cold weather wore on my mom's spirit. She started calling the bad weather in Louisiana "lousyana."

Mom was a progressive woman for those days. The way the culture there treated women bothered her a lot. Women were powerless. Men ran the show. She felt as though time was stuck for sixties-era women in her world, and this fueled her desire to leave for a more progressive place.

Her powers of persuasion worked. By May 1962, our family was in our new home in the college town of Gainesville, Florida. We had done it! We had returned to Florida, where my mother's side of the family lived and where she had been born.

Her very own arrival in this world, unlike mine in a nice hospital, had been much less informal, if not rustic.

Her mother, Doris, had delivered my mom in 1936, with my great-grandfather Dr. Irving P. Philpot attending her—in a barn.

She didn't even have a birth certificate. We guessed that the doctor had gotten too busy to remember to fill one out. He would do the same thing with my mom's brother, Sidney, almost two years later. Granddaddy Philpot had been known for not liking to fill out paperwork.

These had been minor details for a country doctor who made house calls through the northern region of Florida. Back then, there had been no health insurance, much less access to extra money, given that it was during the Great Depression. People had made due with what they had, a far cry from today.

Our lives there, in the rural neck of the woods, were special. I remember one Christmas we were at Nanna and Papaw's house. They had a huge Christmas tree in the center of the living room. It felt like it must have been twenty-five feet high from the ground to the ceiling. A mountain of at least two hundred Christmas presents was underneath its branches, which were covered with red-, blue-, green-, and orange-colored lights and silver icicles. As soon as all of our family members gathered around the tree, my uncle started handing out our presents.

I remember my aunt Elaine's present to me the most. It was a camera and a roll of film. She explained to me how it worked. I was intrigued. It seemed magical. I loaded the camera with film, aimed my camera at family members, and clicked until I couldn't anymore, which meant I was out of film.

Aunt Elaine then showed me how to wind the film back into its container so my mom could drive me to the nearest drugstore to have the film sent to a photo lab to be developed. Within a few days, I would be able to see my results. Pretty exciting, I thought. I began to use my camera as my voice. It was much easier for me to take a picture than to explain. Besides, no one could argue with a photograph, especially then. There was no Photoshop software to edit it, no smartphone filter to make it more perfect.

After my great-granddad passed, my mother would share stories she remembered of watching him work. She showed me his journals where he documented things he had traded with his patients so he would be paid for his services, such as a bushel of oranges and a peck of sweet potatoes.

Mom would also share remedies for headaches and cramps with me that she had learned from him. He loved using sassafras. Sassafras, which is used in making root beer, is an oil once used as a blood thinner, a vasodilator, and a remedy for kidney stones. It was also used back then as an antiseptic and painkiller. Before World War I, research had reportedly shown that people who drank sassafras tea had fewer throat infections and colds.

In the winter, after the first frost, my mom would take me to a field behind the old farm where she was born, where there was a field of sassafras trees. Mom taught me that as the weather turned cold and the plant began to withdraw energy into the earth, it marked the perfect time for harvesting the medicinal roots because the sap goes to the root. We would have a shovel and paper bag in our hands as we made our way through the field. We could safely harvest some of the roots without damaging the tree.

Some family members who knew my mom and I were headed for the sassafras field would jokingly say it was easier to find marijuana growing in the wild than a sassafras tree. My great-granddad had made a note on the side of his journal explaining that paleobotanists said the sassafras is like the ginkgo, a living fossil going back some one hundred million years. They should have stuck a label on the tree: "Caution: eating sassafras may produce cancer in dinosaurs."

This was a family joke about sassafras because one of our ancestors was Elizabeth Philpot. Elizabeth was an early nineteenth-century British fossil collector, amateur paleontologist, and artist who collected fossils from the cliffs around Lyme Regis in Dorset on the southern coast of England.

She is best known today for her collaboration and friendship with the well-known fossil hunter Mary Anning. When Anning discovered that belemnite fossils contained ink sacks, it was Philpot who discovered that the fossilized ink could be revived with water and used for illustrations, which became a common practice for local artists.

I think after hearing my mom share stories about Great-Grandad's work in rural medicine is when I started considering becoming a doctor like him one day. He cared about people. It was not about money. He was a beloved part of the community, and he wanted genuinely to help. I saw that his devotion was the backbone of medicine, and I wanted to be a part of that.

I got a lot of my early spiritual training from my mom. While she might have been known as a housewife, for my sisters, my brother (Tommy), and I, she was our fearless leader and spiritual teacher. Our home was her church. And so were the woods. She taught us how to cook, clean, and play. Mom was Dad's domestic goddess and our domestic drill sergeant.

Our uncles would call her our "domestic engineer." They thought the term *housewife* was demeaning. However, Mom would disagree. She thought it was her holy assignment. She said God gave us each a holy assignment before we were born. I would watch Mom sometimes pray when she felt tired and out of gas. I'd hear her say, "God, please allow me to remember what I promised you I would do before I came to earth for you."

Mom called our bodies our temples. She demanded that we respect them as if they were our suits of armor. Polish them by providing nurturing, healthful foods, and move them in physical activities so they would not get stiff and rusty.

Sometimes we would play outdoor games like football or hide-and-seek. We did not think of it as exercise, but certainly, it got us moving. We would also be active doing manual labor through our chores, like mowing the lawn, raking leaves, sweeping the floor, making the bed, taking out the trash. You know, the things around the house that most kids did back then.

Sometimes kids could earn an allowance for these chores, but nope, not us. However, Mom would sometimes reward us by taking us to the clothing store. If we saw a nice outfit or dress we liked and she knew we needed it, she'd treat us to it for all our hard work.

In the kitchen, she would tell us what constituted a balanced meal. "Think of food like an artist's palette—the more colorful the food on your plate, the more balanced and healthy it is," she'd say, and that, again, was ahead of its time.

I heard my home economics teacher in middle school say the same thing. Yes, when I was thirteen, it was a requirement in middle schools for all students, regardless of gender, to take home economics (where we learned how to cook), agriculture engineering (where we learned how to plant foods we could eat and yes, owing to our rather rural upbringing, how to "ring chickens' necks").

That last activity I could never stomach. I remember calling my mom to come get me from school because I couldn't take watching this beautiful bird who was our teacher's friend become, within seconds, our teacher's dinner for the night. I had vowed to be a skinny farmer from that day forward.

My mother tried teaching us unconditional love. However,

with all these chores we had to do after school and on the weekends, it sometimes was confusing. We knew chores were expected to be completed, and if not, well, it didn't feel like unconditional love coming from her when we failed.

Mom also had the highest of expectations. Failure wasn't an option and neither were poor grades in school. She always wanted us to put our hearts and souls into everything, no matter how small the task appeared. She wanted us to know that every holy assignment was important regardless if someone was a janitor, a doctor, a lawyer, a teacher, or a housekeeper. All jobs were as worthy as the other.

She also taught us that money doesn't buy happiness. Mom wanted us to fully understand her belief about what our souls crave—our connection to God and his holy assignment for us. Each one of us has a different job to do.

She would then caution us to watch out for superficial relationships with things, people, and roles. She told us that, eventually, these relationships would no longer serve our desire to live our truths. It was early wisdom that has served me throughout my life. Her philosophy also helped me to become an independent thinker, which has led me to question modern medicine and the way I view our healthcare system.

I also learned many things from my father, a man who was less comfortable with emotional relationships. We bonded over our joint love of hunting. I even learned how to shoot a gun. I was my dad's little Annie Oakley. Shooting guns is much like shooting a camera except you would never point a gun at anyone unless your life depended on it.

Hunting, for me, was an experience in nature. I enjoyed being out in the open—not killing something. I also liked that I got to get dressed in these camouflage pants, shirt, hats, and tennis shoes. It was a break from wearing a dress to school every day.

I remember that my mom would braid my hair into two pigtails. I called one sugar and the other spice. My hair unbraided was down to the back of my knees. I was my daddy's little girl, his friend in the woods, and this activity also fueled my independent streak. But I also had a feminine side. I was raised to know that I could do anything—dress up, be a girl, or get dirty in the woods. This was empowering.

I was also given a lot of freedom in the woods and learned a lot about wildlife. Birds, deer, bobcats, you name it. The animals became my friends. I would talk to them when my dad wasn't around. When he would walk up on my talking to them, he'd say I was going to scare them off. Dad would teach me how to look for signs and trails and to study animal behaviors as well as how to identify males from females. He had two rules for hunting. One was never to kill the females because they took care of their offspring. The other was only kill what you're gonna eat.

At this point, I wanted to become a vegetarian. I loved animals. I could trust animals more than people. I knew what they would do.

I pretty much hunted and fished my way up until about eleventh grade. This was when my dad thought I was at the age when I needed to spend more time with my mother and do girly kinds of things. I was confused and lost. I didn't want to stop going to the woods with my dad, but I guess I didn't have a choice. I was to obey him.

The 1970s was a decade of social change in the United States, with the civil rights and feminist movements often in the news. The portrayal of family life on television became more diverse. One of our parents' favorite TV shows was *All in the Family*. The show was about working-class families. Dad began to remind my sisters and me of Archie Bunker, the colorful and oft-crude father or paternal character on the show.

Every now and again, if we were good, we'd watch *The Waltons*, a TV show about a close-knit Appalachian clan that provided sentimental portrayals of an ideal nuclear and extended family.

That was not us!

Our family was chaotic at times. Mom's youngest brother, Richard, called us the X-rated Waltons when he came for dinner. We'd cuss and fuss at the dinner table, tell dirty jokes, and be unorthodox. This is who we were—independent-minded and original, traits I still value decades hence.

At this time in my life, graduation was approaching, and I didn't have a clue as to where I was going to college or what I really wanted to do. I was working three jobs while finishing my senior year so I could go to Europe for a student-exchange program.

Our parents taught us to create everything we wanted in life by working and taking care of ourselves—to be self-sufficient. I must have heard "Give a man a fish, and you feed him for a day; teach a man to fish, and you feed him for a lifetime" a thousand times while growing up.

I was accepted into the registered nurse program at Santa Fe Community College, but deep down in my heart, I knew it wasn't what I really wanted to do. I was curious about medical school but didn't know if I was ready or up for such a long road.

In August 1979, I started nursing school. Within a few months, I felt like this just didn't fit. I wanted more. I wasn't feeling satisfied. What I was doing wasn't in alignment with my soul. I dropped out of the nursing program, confident in my decision but clueless about where I was truly meant to be.

I continued going to college under the general-education degree requirements, giving me two more years to declare a major. I started taking math, science, and photography classes. These three subjects came naturally to me. I was also working full time for the local regional newspaper, the *Gainesville Sun*, which was owned at the time by the *New York Times*. I worked as a paste-up artist before pagination and computers took over, helping to build the newspaper that would eventually get printed for local readers.

Within months my photography teacher admired my work. She had shared with me that she was dating the photo chief at the *Gainesville Sun*. His name was Gary. Gary suggested I take a photojournalism class with one of his colleagues, named Carla Hotvedt.

Carla began to mentor me and asked if I wanted to shoot an assignment for the newspaper. I did, and then I was hooked. I loved telling a story with my camera. It was fun! I got to meet incredible people who were like-minded and wanted to discover the truth. Journalists are great "salt-of-the-earth people." Every day was different. My life felt exciting and effortless. I joined the National Press Photographers Association and quickly became an award-winning photographer.

I received my Bachelor of Science degree in photojournalism from the University of Florida and began freelancing for the *Sun* and a variety of newspapers throughout the state. They included the *St. Petersburg* (now *Tampa Bay*) *Times*, the *Fort Lauderdale Sun-Sentinel*, *USA Today*, *Hudson Valley Magazine*, *New Spaces Magazine*, and *New York Magazine*.

I've had the privilege of photographing celebrities such as former UF Gator and NFL great Emmitt Smith, actor Paul Newman, General Norman Schwarzkopf, talk-show host Phil Donahue, country stars Kenny Rogers and Ronnie Milsap, actor-musician River Phoenix, Grammy winner Melanie Safka, and Chris Noth (a.k.a. *Sex* in *the City*'s Mr. Big).

I won national recognition for my work and have exhibited

in galleries and museums in San Francisco, New York, and Miami. I received the Kodak Eastman Impact of Photography award and have been listed in *Who's Who among Women Photojournalists* since the eighties.

Working behind the lens stoked my creative side and also allowed me to do good—to shine a light on those who were powerless, helpless, in need.

However, photojournalism is tough work. You see things you can't unsee. That happened to me in August 1990. At the beginning of the fall semester, five University of Florida college students were brutally slain in separate attacks in off-campus apartments.

On August 27, Christa Hoyt, eighteen, an Alachua County Sheriff's Explorer, was found dead in her southwest Gainesville duplex apartment. She had been decapitated and mutilated, and her body had been posed by the killer. She was the third victim. My father worked with her father. It was a horrific crime that shocked a community.

Covering this story did a number on my head, especially since I grew up in Gainesville. Most of my life, our community was pretty quiet. Some people didn't lock their doors until then. After I finished my assignment on this horrific case, I knew I needed a break from newspaper life. And once again, my focus turned to medicine.

I started working at Shands Teaching Hospital's Learning Resource Center as a medical photographer. Shands is a large medical center affiliated with the University of Florida that serves the North Central Florida region. It was here that I was given the opportunity to do a documentary-photography workshop with Mary Ellen Mark. She was the photojournalist who became known for her work with Mother Teresa.

Mark taught me to use a wide-angle lens to be able to get

into the scenes of my subjects. Using this technique would ensure more emotions in my photographic work. She also shared with me that she, too, thought I was burned out. She also saw that the job I currently had was too repetitious for my style and personality. Mary Ellen praised my work, saying I had a gift of catching my subjects' raw feelings in front of my camera.

Within a few years, my photography position ended, and I took another turn toward a higher calling that continued to knock. I was off to massage school—not to become a massage therapist but to do my prerequisite work for medical school.

Massage school taught me about the body, mind, and spirit connection, much more than what my mother had taught us as children. The balance of all three promotes healthy and happy lives. It also taught me how healing and powerful our hands are, especially when we touch each other in appropriate ways to bring comfort.

I did become a licensed massage therapist, giving me the license "to touch"—and as fate would have it, most of my classmates were from New York.

For most of my life, I was told I should move to New York because I was an Aries, an astrological sign that liked things to happen fast—like in a New York minute.

So just as I thought I had a clear path to medical school, I met Stelli Dounson, a sales manager at Naylor Publications. Dounson invited me to work on her healthcare publications.

As life would have it, I was carried by my destiny to join this company. I hadn't given up on going to medical school, but I thought it would be kind of fun to ride the wave of life and earn some great money for a while. And I did. At Naylor, I more than quadrupled my income as a photojournalist. I was calling on key thought leaders and decision makers at the top pharmaceutical, medical-device, and medical-supply companies in the world.

One day I was talking with the CEO and president of a medical-device company, and he asked if I'd be willing to relocate. He said I needed to move to a territory in the Northeast. He knew I was interested in medical school and claimed that region had some of the best.

Next thing you know, I was offered a position in Westchester County, New York, with a high-risk obstetrics company providing home uterine-activity monitors, Terbutaline, Reglan, Zofran, and insulin through a mini–med pump. Our corporate office was located in Marietta, Georgia.

Mary Etta was my mother's name. I figured it was a good sign. Perhaps this was a clue that I was onto what she had described as my "holy assignment." Besides, I was being offered double what Naylor had offered.

Remember those classmates from massage school? A few of them lived close to where I was moving. I had a few buddies I had stayed in touch with since graduation. So I felt safe in case I got lonely.

I have come to realize that the legacy my parents gave me is something I have used throughout my life to succeed: a strong work ethic and the ability to read people and situations by using my five senses (sight, touch, smell, taste, and hearing) plus one more, trusting my primal instinct, that gut feeling. These six senses supply our brain with information that points in the direction of truth and our divine flow.

I used to think that someone's words and actions had to align to be true. But not anymore. People can be slick, creating the illusion you want to hear or see. I learned to sit still in the moments of my interactions with someone, especially in our introduction to each other or first meeting to be able to feel my gut response. I have found my gut never lies, but people do. So now I look for three things to align in people I bring into my inner circle or heart: actions, words, and how they feel to my gut. This remains the barometer to my heart.

My mom would recite 2 Corinthians 5:7: "For we walk by faith, not by sight."

I keep that within my heart in all that I do—as a daughter, a sister, a friend, a lover, a photojournalist, or a medical-device sales representative. I truly care, and I have come to learn that life is about serving, loving, and doing my best.

That is why I am writing this book—I've learned some things in my healthcare journey that I need to share with all women and all men. I think they are life-changing.

Chapter 3

The View from the Inside

I began my career in medical-device sales with a high-risk obstetrics company in 1998.

It was a huge learning curve, but I was getting an education about more than simply medical devices. I was getting a front-row seat to our healthcare system, which has changed mightily in the two decades hence.

My first training was in the world of high-risk obstetrics.

Keep in mind that during this time, companies did not give out laptop computers the way they do today. Neither did we have smartphones or GPS devices. I was handed five three-inch-thick ring binders with loads of Xerox copies of clinical information on hyperemesis, high blood pressure, preeclampsia, gestational diabetes, and preterm labor.

I had to learn this detailed medical information in two weeks.

You can imagine the mixed emotions and thoughts running through my head. Wow! Two weeks, when most obstetrics residents have four years. I felt fortunate, excited, and anxious all at once. As an account executive, I would be responsible for educating and promoting our portfolio of products to physicians, nurses, case managers, and discharge planners for our high-risk obstetrics company in and out of the hospital.

My teammates in the medical industry lovingly compare

the training required to sell medical devices, medical supplies, or pharmaceutical products like going to a medical boot camp. It's intense, grueling, and the longest two weeks away from home to say the least. Lots of scientific and clinical information to learn and be tested on in a very short period. Oral and written exams are given to us very much like those given to physicians when they are trying to become board certified. A 90 percent or better is expected by our company. Anything less, and you can be sent home with no future in the organization, depending on the company.

We had to be quick studies, to learn all there was to know about the disease state so we could go toe to toe with physicians about why they should use our products to improve patient outcomes and quality of life. In training, we also learned about covered payers (insurance companies who covered our services) as well as how to handle the total office call—getting to know everyone in the physician's office and the roles they played.

We operated on the premise that everyone in the office and the hospital is a valuable person and has a function in patient care. It starts the moment the phone rings to book an appointment and lasts until the patient is discharged (no longer needing services from them).

I studied hard. I was determined, and I passed.

My territory was large. It covered five counties (Westchester, Dutchess, Orange, Rockland, and Putnam) upstate from New York City—also known as "the city" to New Yorkers, as if there is no other city. This meant I had to purchase an Upstate New York atlas to find my call points, physicians' offices, clinics, and hospitals.

Up until now, I hadn't given too much thought to the business of bringing babies into the world. I thought giving birth was a natural progression in life, without risk, and was pretty easy. Right? Well, at least in my family. Interestingly enough I was thirty-seven years old. Not that I was thinking about having a baby, but my recruiter and I joked about how it took me nine months to create my job at the high-obstetrics company. I quickly learned not every woman is so lucky.

Since obstetrics has no "on-label" medications or products with indications, everything is off-label. The reason for no on-label products is that obstetricians are sued the most out of any other specialty. Perhaps this is because they are also the only specialty responsible for a life from conception until eighteen years of age.

Our industry lies in the middle of any legal conundrum. The thought is that if you sue the doctor, then you will sue the company responsible for the products they use.

Obstetrics is also responsible for the highest cost in healthcare. To get around this minor detail, I had to demonstrate the safety and efficacy of our products. I achieved this by going over the clinical studies with physicians and hospitals, proving it was a safe product to use. I also demonstrated our products would aid in prolonging the patient's pregnancy.

Video recording and role-playing were used a lot to simulate a real live call. We each had to give a twenty-minute in-service to our peers, pretending they were the hospital staff. Within the presentations, we had to identify the appropriate patients and demonstrate how to apply our device and review dosing.

We learned how to identify multiple risk factors for patients who are appropriate. Among those risk factors were advanced maternal age (over thirty-five) and medical conditions before pregnancy (e.g., high blood pressure; lung, kidney, or heart problems; diabetes; autoimmune disease; sexually transmitted diseases [STDs]; or chronic infections such as human immunodeficiency virus [HIV]).

It was a crash course in obstetrics but fascinating nonetheless, which added to the rewarding aspect of this career choice/endeavor.

It also presented great challenges. I had to be resilient and persistent throughout the entire day as a great deal of effort is required to see an ob-gyn or perinatologist or nurse, especially in the beginning of a relationship that has not already been established. I was starting anew in every respect.

My days were super long, beginning around 5:00 a.m. and ending around 11:00 p.m. I spent a lot of time in my car learning the geography of my territory. The bonus to all of my car time was that my area was stunningly beautiful. I got to see the Hudson River and Bear Mountain daily, even as I was driving 750 miles or so a week, earning the nickname "road warrior" from my sisters.

As a part of my storytelling, to help develop and personalize my working relationships in a tough field, I would let nurses and physicians know I had relocated from Gainesville, Florida.

They would all shake their heads and ask why would I leave all that warm weather and sunshine. People were gracious and friendly. Many would invite me out to eat and offer to show me around. I did not feel like a southerner or outsider for long.

Nancy Kirshenbaum, MD, ob-gyn, MFM, my highest-volume prescriber, would always keep me in check with my clinical information when I would go toe to toe with her in reviewing studies. She was one of my best teachers in the field and became a great friend. I always knew when I heard her ask, "So, which medical school did you go to again, and how many patients are you treating?" that it was time to take a step back and listen, rather than sell.

There was a lot of independence in my job, which I loved. Every day was different and exciting in its own way. I had to stay organized and plan my days explicitly, but that taught me dedication.

I learned along the way that nurses are the best resources in the hospital. Ask any resident who knows what's going on with his or her patients, and he or she will tell you to ask the nurse, but don't piss him or her off because then you've cut your arm off for good.

One day at Westchester Medical Center, a labor and delivery patient found out through my housemate that I had been a photojournalist and invited me to photograph her birth, so I did, harkening back to my days behind the camera but enjoying this opportunity to be creative nonetheless.

Although most of my duties as a sales rep may not have been quite as glamorous, I was rarely bored and met great people who became my New York family.

I loved my work. It required the best of me—taking on the pressure of closing sales and smiling all day and then coming home at nights and often on weekends to tend to mounds of paperwork. I began to enjoy the flow of the organization and the finesse involved when I'd completed my week, putting the final touches on the required reports.

I could then kick back and relax, knowing that I had helped my physician and hospital accounts deliver healthy and happy babies. That meant something, to be a part of the healthcare process that gave new mothers their dreams.

In short, I got to witness a lot of miracles. On the other hand, I was able to learn a lot of eye-opening and unpleasant facts about our healthcare system.

Among my early observations: I saw many doctors' hands being tied and patient care being delayed by insurance-company tactics, denying services and creating an appeals process. This created more work for physicians to get the plan of care they wanted to be approved for their patients. The tail indeed wagged the dog. But that analogy is hardly funny because people's lives were at stake.

The runaround often led to some significantly bad outcomes, for which the physician was later held accountable through lawsuits. All because an insurance company did not want to deliver the care owed to its contracted patient.

But that is just the tip of the iceberg as our medical system falls apart, as care is denied, providers disband, and more doctors leave because they are pawns in a huge and deepening mess.

How would you fare if you got caught in the middle of it through no fault of your own?

This is why I want to share my insider view—so you fully understand what we are dealing with. A giant, unwieldy system that has made healthcare impersonal and careless.

We need all the information about our healthcare system so we can prepare ourselves to be actively engaged and can control our own care.

Chapter 4
Paralysis by Analysis

In June 2017, after finishing my rounds at Greenwich Hospital, I felt tired and thought another cup of coffee might boost my energy.

As I walked up two flights of stairs, I got to the top and noticed not far from the coffee machine a man chatting with a beautiful woman. Upon first glance, I thought she looked familiar, but I also thought I was probably daydreaming or weary from not sleeping well the night before. After all, working in healthcare now makes for a long workday and short, restless nights.

Suddenly, the woman's eyes and mine locked, and within a few seconds, she started to scream my name. "Shary Connella!" she squealed. I responded right back: "Kaye Jimenez!"

Kaye was my first sales manager at the high-risk obstetrics company where I had worked. I hadn't seen her in about sixteen years. We were both so overjoyed to see each other that we kept giving each other bear hugs as we teared up laughing at life's synchronicity.

It wasn't long before we began to share all the changes in healthcare since our journeys had taken us in different directions with other companies.

As it turned out, we were thinking the same thing: paralysis by analysis. That is the term we use when talking about reimbursement and insurance companies or payers. And for us, this is the most impactful piece of our broken healthcare system. It has changed the destiny of our healthcare system dating back to 1973. It either slows down treatment or prevents us from treatment. And it has continued to get worse.

"So, Shar, what do you think you learned in the last two decades working in the healthcare industry as a sales representative?" she asked.

I replied that I know it is a labor of love and an act of service. But on the other side, we both agreed that the Affordable Healthcare Act, better known as Obamacare, continues to have a negative impact on patients' lives.

It's just a matter of time before the whole system comes crashing down, even as a new Congress and administration try to do damage control and fix a flawed plan that seemed destined to implode from the start.

When I traveled to India six years ago, I remember my Indian doctor friends telling me to make sure I checked with the Centers for Disease Control and Prevention before I traveled and to take all precautions before leaving. They warned that I didn't want to end up in the hospital over there because I could come out with something far worse than before I went in.

It's funny—now I tell people here to be careful if you are admitted to the hospital in the United States because you could come out with something far worse than when you went in, like MRSA (methicillin-resistant Staphylococcus aureus).

I see this all the time in hospitals. It is a scary and a real thing.

As I take stock of where we are now in healthcare, I look back on my days at the high-risk obstetrics company and what surely were the beginnings of the nosedive in our system. It didn't just happen overnight.

I watched physicians work like artists when they approached their patients' healthcare. Physicians had enough time to spend with them, combining wisdom, knowledge, and intuition as their preferred tools in the medicine bag, using traditional and controversial methods to help women bring a baby to full term, thirty-seven weeks.

What I also saw was this: most physicians were not good business professionals. They wanted to focus on patient care, not paperwork or billing. However, this new system has become so convoluted, they are now trapped in treating and compliance with new regulations and demands created by the healthcare law.

The amount of paperwork insurance companies requires physicians to fill out now, with clinical documentation for services or products for a patient, is ridiculous and time consuming. This protocol by insurance companies is a waste of physicians' time and prevents doctors from spending more time with patients. Perhaps this is why patients are no longer being diagnosed accurately in a timely manner. This may actually cost the insurance companies more money in the long run because more aggressive treatments may be needed to ensure better outcomes.

Back when I first started, I knew there were two camps as far as high-risk pregnancy was concerned. One school of thought believed tocolytic drugs worked to stop preterm delivery, and one didn't. Unless you had the inside scoop or education to give you the confidence to challenge your physician by asking questions, you could end up in the camp who didn't use tocolytics, and deliver your baby too soon.

Tocolytic drugs are medications that can inhibit labor and slow down or halt the contractions of the uterus. Today they are widely used to treat premature labor and permit pregnancy to proceed so the fetus can gain in size and maturity before being born.

Terbutaline was a tocolytic commonly used then, even when most specialists were not sure of the side effects to the fetus when administered to the mother. Terbutaline pump therapy was what I promoted at the high-risk obstetrics company. I had one of the top prescribers in the country for terbutaline pump therapy, Dr. Rich Viscarello.

Women from all over the world would fly into Stamford, Connecticut, to have their pregnancies managed by Dr. Viscarello.

In 2001, I helped him with a study looking at the safety and efficacy of terbutaline pump therapy and twin pregnancies. Despite all the clinical studies we had on terbutaline pump therapy, every now and then an insurance company would slap a physician on the wrist by denying its usage, slowing down a physician and requiring more clinical documentation or a letter of appeal.

This was maddening for both me and the physicians. Unfortunately, I witnessed several pregnant patients who were denied terbutaline pump therapy go into preterm labor, delivering too early. This created birth defects like premature lungs, resulting in higher costs and a lifetime of dealing with chronic respiratory issues. It all could have been prevented if insurance providers hadn't gotten in the way of science and care.

In 2003 I joined a cardiovascular pharmaceutical company. Wow, was this job ever an eye-opener. I got to see that some physicians were prescribing cardiovascular medicine based on what a pharmaceutical company could do for their personal needs, not the needs or the best interests of their patients' safety.

For example, as an option, if someone had high triglycerides, our pharmaceutical company would offer the first FDA-approved fish oil, prescribed under the name Lovaza. This medication was covered first tier (lowest co-pay available) on most insurance plans, but doctors would prescribe Niaspan instead because of incentives from the drug company, including trips, money, or paid speaking engagements.

Niaspan had horrible side effects, such as feeling like you might pass out; fast, pounding, or uneven heartbeats; feeling short of breath; swelling; and flushing so bad that patients would experience feeling like their chest was on fire—whereas Lovaza's biggest side effect was burping.

In 2010, along with the new Obamacare program, lawmakers also passed the Physician Payments Sunshine Act. It was created to increase transparency of financial relationships between healthcare providers and pharmaceutical manufacturers and to uncover potential conflicts of interest.

The Sunshine Act requires manufacturers of drugs, medical devices, and biological and medical supplies covered by the three federal healthcare programs—Medicare, Medicaid, and State Children's Health Insurance Program—to collect and track all financial relationships with physicians and teaching hospitals and to report these data to the Centers for Medicare and Medicaid Services.

The act examines the financial relationships between physicians and medical-product manufacturers, which are common and can include everything from free meals to consulting or speaker fees and direct research funding.

On the surface, these relationships can have many positive outcomes—particularly in the context of consulting and research funding—and are often a key component in the development of new drugs and devices.

However, they can also create conflicts of interest, and in some cases, they can blur the line between promotional activities and the conduct of medical research, training, and practice.

A 2009 nationwide survey by the Institute of Medicine in Washington, DC, found that nearly 84 percent of physicians had some form of financial interaction with manufacturers of drugs, devices, biologicals, and medical supplies. The survey discovered most of these interactions were meals provided in offices or clinical settings.

The survey also uncovered that about 20 percent of these physicians received reimbursements for attending meetings or continuing-medical-education events. Less than 15 percent of these physicians received payments for professional services. These percentages were notably lower than found in a similar survey five years earlier.

A number of factors likely contributed to this decrease, including changes within the pharmaceutical industry driven by the financial crisis, leading to reducing sales-force staffing and shifting marketing strategies.

The Sunshine Act marked a thin attempt by politicians to expose drug-manufacturer kickbacks in the medical profession, although as far as anyone can tell, it's done little if anything to inspire real change. The hand greasing continues.

So, while medical offices were enjoying the largesse of drug and medical product reps, patients were getting shortchanged on their own small but crucial perks.

Before I left the cardiovascular pharmaceutical company, some medical offices started to eliminate drug samples, preventing patients from a seven-day supply and claiming it was an incentive for doctors to write medicines for a particular drug company. This could not have been further from the truth. Samples were designed for physicians to give to patients to see if they could tolerate a medication before purchasing a thirty-day supply. Most patients will know within three days if they can tolerate it or not without investing any money—and in some cases, such investments were significant.

In addition to the Sunshine Act, the Stark Law was created to prohibit physician self-referral, specifically a referral by a physician of a Medicare or Medicaid patient to an entity providing designated health services. If the physician (or an immediate family member) has a financial relationship with that entity, they are in violation of the Stark Law.

The Sunshine Act and the Stark Law have spooked so many physicians, so much so that some have stopped giving samples to their patients amid fears that it could be seen as an incentive influencing them to write a prescription.

Take, for example, one of my family friends, Joanne. She is seventy-six and a diabetic. She and her husband were living on a fixed income, barely able to pay living expenses due to their illnesses. They were diagnosed with diabetes in their early sixties, and like most of us, neither had planned on having to navigate a significant medical condition so early in life. They imagined living together pretty healthily well into their nineties.

Joanne was on eleven medications. For a patient who is not on more than one medication, like a diabetic, this doesn't seem like a big deal, right? However, if you are like Joanne or her husband, you could be on at least five or more medications with a sixty-dollar-or-more co-pay for each prescription to be filled. Do the math. If you're a retired diabetic like Joanne and her husband, this could become a financial burden very quickly.

Imagine that you are on eleven or more meds, and you do

not get a sample to try. You fill your thirty-day prescription, and then you cannot tolerate it because you have started to experience side effects. You just blew sixty dollars and have to go back to the doctor to find an alternative medication—and likely pay to fill that. This expense could have been avoided if the patient's doctor gave you samples first.

Remember the medical mandate "First, do no harm" ("*Primum nonnocere*")? It is a part of the Hippocratic oath. I have to wonder if some of today's doctors even think about the harm they are doing by loading up patients with prescriptions and not asking if the cost could be a burden.

If you can't afford good food or struggle to pay the electric bill, should you be forced to pay $400 in co-pays while your physicians do some experimenting on what works best for you? We have to change this formula.

I've watched several friends struggle with this issue.

My childhood pal Cindy has experienced similar frustrations to Joanne; however, hers are for a different diagnosis—anxiety and depression, which are mental health concerns.

Cindy had been asking me about the hidden dangers of benzodiazepine use. I have never worked in the arena or modality of mental healthcare. However, I could easily surf the internet and do a little research as well as, ask the primary care physicians I know for their thoughts on her situation.

I discovered that Xanax, Ativan, and Valium are probably the most common short- and long-acting benzodiazepines used.

Almost three decades after a pundit penned the assertion, "America is still a Xanax nation," it remains the most popular psychiatric drug. It continues to top more recently introduced medicines like the sleeping pill Ambien (number two) and the antidepressant Lexapro (number three). Doctors write nearly fifty million prescriptions for Xanax, or alprazolam (the cheap, generic equivalent), every year. That's more than one Xanax prescription written every second, according to the medical publication *JAMA Psychiatry*.

Xanax hit the market in 1981. Before it, Valium was the most popular drug in America for most of the seventies. I also learned that in the last year, there have been several studies/stories about the risks associated with benzodiazepine abuse. And while benzodiazepines have been prescribed for decades to treat anxiety and seizure disorders, as well as insomnia, the possible threat of overusing them is real, and with that comes dependency, overdose, and the potential of death.

Did you know that since 2010, there have been 6,507 US drug-overdose deaths that were known to have involved benzodiazepines?

"Overdose rose at a faster rate than prescriptions, suggesting that people were using benzodiazepines in a riskier way over time," Dr. Marcus, assistant professor of medicine at Albert Einstein College of Medicine in New York, told *Health* magazine in a February 2016 article.

"Benzodiazepine prescriptions are widespread, but their use may not be the smart choice for many patients," he warned.

For Cindy, there were significant repercussions for her antianxiety medication use. Doctors failed to address her concerns about other health issues, blaming her symptoms on these medications and their overuse.

One day Cindy, who was sixty-five at the time, called me in hysterics, claiming she couldn't breathe. She thought she was having a heart attack. So she called 911, and an ambulance took her to the local hospital.

Cindy arrived at the ER with a myriad of symptoms associated with Xanax use—which can mimic a heart attack—

including shortness of breath, chest pains, labored breathing, and dizziness.

Withdrawal symptoms from Xanax use are also similar—adding heart palpitations and high blood pressure to the mix.

Cindy, who presented with these symptoms, turned over her Obamacare insurance card. Once the ER healthcare professional discovered she was on anti-anxiety medications and what her insurance coverage was, Cindy said she was immediately disconnected from oxygen and was prepared for transport to a mental health facility across town.

Refusing to check her physical symptoms any further for signs of a cardiac problem, the healthcare team insisted her anxiety caused her shortness of breath and chest pains. The team then invoked Florida's Baker Act statute and sent her for three days to the mental health facility—the legal limit for forcing her to stay. The physicians there wrote her more antianxiety prescriptions and then discharged her to go home.

Five years prior, Cindy said she had gone to her primary care physician for a yearly checkup. After the doctor had taken her vital signs, he had asked her how things were going. She had shared that her work had been stressful. Her physician had then asked if she had been working with a professional counselor to manage her stress. Cindy had replied very quickly, yes. But she had added that talk therapy hadn't worked well for her. The physician had then recommended that she take Xanax.

As hard as it is to believe, Cindy contends her physician had not explained to her that benzodiazepines are highly addictive and regarded by some as harder to quit than heroin. Apparently, the physician had failed to review the side effect profile warning Cindy of the severity of getting hooked on this medication and the difficulty to stop.

The side effects of taking benzodiazepine had kicked in, no longer giving Cindy the relief she once received when she first began taking Xanax.

Cindy shared a story with me that she had read about Fleetwood Mac's Steve Nicks's one-time addiction to Klonopin, which is in the Valium family. Nicks had to be hospitalized to heal her addiction. Cindy claims Nicks had the money to be hospitalized when her own insurance wouldn't pay. But Cindy doesn't.

Now, Cindy is on an unstable path, living alone in a very remote and secluded area of North Central Florida, scared to drive her truck because she is afraid she could kill someone while driving under the influence of her medication. She refuses to drive to doctor's appointments or for medical tests. The ER is her only hope of finding out her body's other medical mysteries.

Cindy is convinced there is more happening inside her body other than side effects or withdrawal symptoms from her prescribed medications. Thirty-one physicians later and over forty-five prescribed medications taken, Cindy's health is worsening. She's losing hope that she will ever thrive again. She is feeling like a prisoner in her own world.

I could hear the desperation in her voice—so out of character for Cindy. Most of her life she took care of everyone else. Her house was immaculate. She used to be a runner and bike rider. And now she sits paralyzed in her room—wanting to be alone, feeling ashamed of how she looks.

She keeps asking why. "Why didn't anyone tell me these drugs would do this to me? I would have never taken them."

Her situation has broken my heart. I came home from work two days later to hear Cindy's voice crying on my answering machine. She experienced chest pains and labored breathing again as well as shortness of breath. She kept asking me why no one in the ER had run tests to see if she was having a heart attack or if there was something else wrong?

She called 911 again. The ambulance picked her up again and took her to the ER. When she returned to the ER again, they refused to treat her, saying it was only her anxiety. Cindy begged them to order a blood test, an EKG, and an MRI to see what was going on.

Again, she was denied care and sent to the mental facility. The healthcare professionals at the facility told her she had to go to a specialist outside of the hospital to have the tests done. They explained that the hospital would not do that for her with her type of insurance.

Cindy is now feeling like our system has failed her. She is not alone. The over-prescription of benzodiazepines in older Americans has become a pattern around the nation.

I see this on a daily basis when I round at the hospital. There are many patients waiting to be seen complaining of side effects from Xanax and other benzodiazepines. One study suggests that there are more than 1 billion antidepressants and 3.3 billion antianxiety prescriptions written every year.

There are also many studies published looking at the injuries and medical costs associated with long-term and inappropriate use of benzodiazepines, especially in the elderly population.

Apparently "Mother's Little Helper" is now a good friend of Grandma and Grandpa too.

After spending hours surfing the internet to learn more, I got an email from Marianne Williamson announcing that her latest book, *Tears to Triumph*, which would become a *New York Times* bestseller, was now available in paperback. As I read her email, I saw that her book cover states, "Spiritual

Healing for the Modern Plagues of Anxiety and Depression."

Hmm, I thought. The very two things I had been researching for Cindy.

Marianne wrote:

Dear Friends,

We're living in dramatic times, with a stress on many of our external systems ranging from political to financial to environmental. And not only the outer world is experiencing crisis; internally, we're absorbing the stress as well. We often find ourselves experiencing emotional and psychological anxiety that mirrors the upset of these extraordinary times.

As it says in "A Course in Miracles (ACIM)," we think we have many different problems but we really only have one: our separation from God. That is why I wrote my latest book. My goal was to articulate the spiritual principles that deliver us to inner peace regardless of the conflicts or anxieties of our material circumstances. "Tears to Triumph" articulates spiritual keys to navigating painful times. These keys are drawn from the great religious and spiritual traditions of the world, from the illuminations of Buddha to Moses to Jesus. In the midst of our deepest emotional crises, the inner Light of God is key to our capacity to move beyond the darkness."

Could this be a sign for Cindy, offering her an alternative for healing her anxiety and depression?

I thought to myself that perhaps traditional medicine should reconsider a spiritual component as part of the care for stress and anxiety. But then again, that sort of protocol might stem drug profits and kickbacks. Those are likely too enticing to allow them to stop.

Just thinking about this makes my blood boil. But there are plenty more reasons for my concern.

Shortly after leaving the high-risk obstetrics company, I witnessed another troubling incident that marked yet another sign that our medical system was falling apart. I saw United Hospital, near Rye, New York, close its doors because the wealthy board members who lived in this affluent area did not want to share the hospital with the growing group of Hispanic immigrants in Port Chester, a neighboring city, who used it too.

No one said this was the reason, and you could not prove it. But that was the word—from nurses and others who worked there. The hospital had become a repository for poor people in a place where the rich had always ruled.

I am no stranger to this undercurrent of discrimination and divide.

After moving to this area of New York, I rented a two-bedroom apartment in an old Victorian, on the third floor. I loved being able to see views of the Long Island Sound outside my living room window. I also enjoyed the diversity of my neighborhood. As a southerner, I sometimes felt like an outsider at the beginning of my move, but it was beautiful living among people from different cultures. On the right of my house was a lovely family from China, and on the left a Hispanic family from Mexico. They both were hard working and kept their homes looking immaculate.

United Hospital was blocks from our homes, and I used to call on this medical center when I worked for the high-risk-pregnancy company.

During this era, most hospitals that closed were in

struggling communities with many immigrants. Governor Pataki had announced that New York could no longer support hospitals that were not profitable, and, of course, the ones that served our most vulnerable patients were the first to be shuttered.

The number of Hispanic residents in Port Chester, which has a population of 28,000, had ballooned in recent years. Their numbers had risen from 16 percent in 1980 to 46 percent in 2000.

United Hospital officials contended that 49 percent of patients they saw were on Medicare and 23 percent on Medicaid. This created a financial strain, causing the hospital to close after serving the community since 1889.

However, many of my neighbors thought the real truth was that the wealthy residents of Rye and RyeBrook did not want to be near a Hispanic patient while waiting for care.

Some of my neighbors were nurses working in United's ER. They said they could tell by the disgruntled looks on many of the ER patients from Rye and RyeBrook that being around poor immigrants and Medicaid patients made them uncomfortable. They were more than happy to see the hospital close as they had the means to go to a hospital just three miles away in wealthy Greenwich, Connecticut.

This was when it became truly evident to me that quality healthcare would only be affordable for the wealthy in our country. That is where we are headed. If you can pay for treatment, great. If you rely on insurance and government to protect you, forget it.

Keep in mind that this hospital closed in 2005, five years before Obamacare and the Affordable Care Act became law. I knew then our healthcare system would no longer be affordable for the masses as those with wealth could control care. And Obamacare, as well-meaning as some contend it was, turned our healthcare system into a house of cards.

Yes, more people got coverage. But everyone's coverage, for the most part, got exponentially worse—and for many, way more expensive without an increase in benefits.

Would it be fair to say that in the United States, healthcare is a business? Of course it is.

What is the purpose of any business? Ideally, it is to help and serve the customer. And by "help and serve," I mean to give the customer what he or she needs to resolve his or her concern and to educate him or her on how to change his or her behavior to make sure the concern does not come back.

Many businesses do not practice that form of business strategy (i.e., help and serve). The business of healthcare is no different. All businesses, if they are to survive, must be focused on profit and repeat business. The business of medicine has become more about profits and repeated service and less about true help.

Please appreciate that when I say "true" help, I am talking about giving back control to the person with the problem— the patient. All patients. And since we will all be a patient at one point or another in our lives, it becomes important to understand how to do this.

We can no longer be a health pessimist while waiting for conditions to get worse. We must all come to understand that the business of being a healthcare insurer is to make a profit.

Here's how it works. Insurance companies have this game, making everyone jump through their hurdles. They claim they are going to cover our costs for care, but then they keep healthcare providers from being able to take care of us— making our doctors jump through hoops to get them to pay for the coverage that doctors determine that we need.

Insurance companies are keeping physicians from giving us the care that they've been trained to give. Even as these physicians have passed grueling oral and written tests called boards to prove their competency, payers will deny coverage for their patients.

Yes, these highly trained doctors are being thwarted by having someone who has never been to medical school or has no medical knowledge (or often, a medical director who is no longer treating patients or actively practicing medicine) make decisions for the insurance company on your claims.

I am also hearing from nurses who take care of patients that have to work with an insurance company on a daily basis say that insurance companies have empowered employees with no medical knowledge and only a high school diploma to approve or deny patient claims.

In effect, insurance companies work to keep you from the care that you need. While patients suffer, they engage in things like prolonging your treatment by asking doctors for a letter of medical necessity or asking for a peer-to-peer review of your case. In the time all of this stalling takes place, your condition may get worse. In the end—as sad as it sounds—it is your life versus their profits.

Let's look at another factor driving higher cost in healthcare premiums: lawsuits. America is the most litigious country in the world. In 2016, 512,000 tort law cases were filed in the United States. The cost of these civil lawsuits to our country: $239 billion.

Aware of the heightened legal scrutiny of medicine, physicians must cover all of their bases. To that end, they often order expensive tests that are clinically inappropriate to cover their liability. A positive test result will cause patients to come for continuous treatment. Say you have a health issue, and you're a perfect patient for treatment. This helps to provide profits for your insurer. And all of those records for treatment are kept and tracked.

The business model of being a doctor, for many, has become treating "symptoms," a sort of trial remedy before understanding the underlying cause. And it is OK because if that "try" does not improve your condition, doctors have another "try" or strategy to use.

I've seen this up close. This is why as the patient, you have to be engaged in your healthcare; otherwise, you may experience the "try" scenarios. Sometimes, the first "try" requires a second support to make the first "try" more effective or less problematic in the form of "side effects." And when all the "trying" does not seem to handle the concern, and the problem becomes worse (like all problems do when they are not being properly addressed), it is OK because now the medical system can offer you a more substantial treatment called surgery.

And with the surgery comes recovery that requires more treatment, possibly more medication, and perhaps more surgery if the first "try" of surgery did not turn out as planned.

This ongoing triangulation ensures that the business of medicine is truly a business that is profitable—profitable for the labs that run the lab work, profitable for the technology companies that make the machines, profitable for the pharmaceutical companies that create the medicines, and somehow, believe it or not, profitable for the insurance companies that cover some, most, or all of the treatment and procedures.

How is it possible that all of these businesses are making profits if they are there to support the health and well-being of the people they serve? Sure, they are entitled to make a profit, but at what expense to you as the patient? Is our current business model for medicine being applied appropriately?

Most of us question our healthcare system. And with that, many of us wonder how it could improve if the government continues to get more involved given the government's track record of inaction, obfuscation, and yes, I'll say it, lies.

If you like your health insurance plan, you can keep it. Remember that lie? It was told by President Obama and his supporters as they quickly moved to pass a universal-coverage plan.

But few could keep their plan. Only some were able to keep their doctors. The government did harm, and the system began to unravel, all while lawmakers touted its profundity.

Healthcare officials will tell you that government regulations require scrutinizing the profit-and-loss statements of all of these entities making money off your illness. They will even tell you that they are creating "fee schedules" appropriate for the different procedures, deciding what will be paid and what is considered "reasonable and customary."

In doing so, they are "standardizing" procedures and protocols designed to make everyone the same—one office, facility, or hospital to another. This is the one-size-fits-all mentality. And this will again create more problems within whatever future system they roll out in place of the current one that is falling apart.

What I know for sure: one size does not fit all, and we all know it.

The system itself *is* the problem. The perspective that one size fits all does not work when you are dealing with individuals who don't adhere to the "solution."

That is why, after nearly one hundred years of medicine, countless dollars spent on research, development, and implementation of different "theories" of care, hundreds of foundations, societies, and organizations to create more awareness of the latest disease expected to hit our society, and all the energy and effort aimed at this big machine, our healthcare system has not yielded any true solutions.

I watch with a suspicious side-eye all the celebrities getting on television, the radio, and the internet, appearing in print ads, asking you to "donate" to the latest cause. It has led me to ask one simple question: when did doing the same thing over and over again and expecting different results become the means to an end?

This has not and never will lead to a true solution. Why? Because too many people from too many agencies are making too much money keeping you sick by coming up with fake solutions to problems they continuously look at from the wrong perspective.

Who can you trust for your healthcare?

Let me be blunt: not the president, not hospitals, not your insurance provider.

The person you should be relying on in this is *you*.

Chapter 5

A Snakebite and Sticker Shock

I want to talk about venomous snakes. And no, I'm not alluding to healthcare providers who refuse to pay for treatments. I'm talking about slithering, scary, dangerous reptiles that live around us.

The word *venomous* means that each of these kinds of snakes possesses venom that can cause serious illness, injury, or even death. In North Carolina, one of the worst is the copperhead.

The copperhead is a pit viper. This means it has a sensory pit located midway between the eye and nostril, on either side of its face. The copperhead uses these pits to detect warm-blooded prey.

The copperhead is a relatively small snake, with adults averaging less than three feet (thirty-six inches) in length. This snake has a pale-tan or pinkish-tan background color that darkens toward the midbody area. It has a series of darker crossbands on its outside skin.

While it is certainly dangerous, copperheads do not account for very many human fatalities. It is true—a copperhead bite can do a lot of tissue damage in the area of the bite, but it rarely causes death. With proper medical treatment, there is a good chance a human will survive a bite from this species. But you still need to treat these animals with respect and distance.

So by now, you are probably wondering why I am talking about copperhead snakes in North Carolina. It's because of a cool September night when my sister Tammy realized, after getting ready for bed, that she had forgotten to get her page-turner book out of her truck before falling asleep.

Barefoot and without even thinking to put shoes on first, at approximately 11:00 p.m., she ran downstairs, headed for her truck in her garage. The light was dim on her front porch. As her second foot crossed the threshold of the front door to the house, something grabbed hold of the top of her foot. She let out a scream for Dale.

Quickly, Tammy's leg began to swell to ten times its normal size. Her legs felt like a thousand fire ants had bitten her. As my brother-in-law came to her aid, Tammy told him she thought she had been bitten by a snake.

Dale immediately scanned the front yard in front of the porch with his flashlight. "Yep," he said. "It's a snake, all right. It's a copperhead." He quickly grabbed a shovel to kill the snake and placed it in a bag.

The snake had apparently crawled onto the cool marble tiles to rest outside the front door entrance next to the threshold. As Tammy had exited her house, she had unknowingly disturbed the snake by walking over him.

Dale and Tammy managed to get her inside her truck and headed to the hospital.

Just after being whisked into the ER, during the first few moments of Tammy's emergency care, an insurance co-payment was requested from her husband. Since they were in the midst of her emergency examination, they were both somewhat stunned by the timing.

But of course, without question, Dale paid those fees immediately to avoid any other unnecessary interruptions while Tammy was receiving a medical assessment. It was only after they paid the hospital $300 that the medical team was able to devote its full attention to what was occurring around Tammy.

Following the initial flurry of activity, the doctors recommended Tammy forgo an antivenin treatment and then she was checked periodically for about three to four hours.

The copperhead experts, Dr. Christine Murphy and Dr. William Kerns, medical-toxicology physicians in the emergency department at Carolinas Medical Center, were called in. He even had Tammy sign a form consenting to be in a copperhead-bite study.

"It's a good idea to seek medical attention for any snake bite. It is sometimes hard to tell if you have been bitten by a venomous snake. Some copperhead bites are dry bites with no envenomation," Murphy told the couple.

She said doctors would monitor the bite to see if pain and swelling in the bitten area started spreading to other areas. Sometimes a blood test is performed to identify increased bleeding risk as snake venom can interfere with blood clotting.

If needed, a copperhead bite patient would receive CroFab, an antivenin medication. On some occasions, several doses are required, and a patient may need to be hospitalized for several days.

For Tammy, the examination of the snake bite included checking her vital signs, measuring the wounded area to monitor swelling, a sedative, blood tests, and a tetanus vaccination.

In general, the bulk of her stay was spent marking time or being transferred to one of the three different areas described above. In fact, decisions made to relocate her were primarily to create space for new ER patients, not because Tammy's medical condition had changed.

Those final few hours of waiting occurred in a space that was depressingly small and somewhat run-down. It was larger than a walk-in closet, but it did not have either a window or a private toilet area. The room had a hospital bed and a view of a portable potty that pulled out of an old base cabinet.

Tammy was then moved to an adjacent holding area for another three hours or so and then later moved to yet another small room in the ER area until she received the doctor's clearance to leave.

Keep in mind, throughout this process, she was never advised of any decrease in urgency related to her care or, more specifically, of any changes that would occur relative to the billing structure and financial obligations of her venomous-snakebite wound.

Around 7:00 a.m., Tammy was discharged. She would spend many days with a swollen leg on which she could not walk. When she changed positions from horizontal to vertical, the blood flow changed, causing her leg to swell again. Being the fast study she was, she figured out a way to scoot across the floor from room to room until, finally, the venom worked its way out of her body's system.

But the real wound was just starting. Just as Tammy thought that her snakebite was healed, and just when she thought the whole episode was over, she received a bill for her hospital visit.

Tammy and Dale thought the $300 they paid in the beginning had covered all their responsibilities, as explained by the hospital employee handling their insurance.

Remember that Tammy was moved from the ER to the observation room? Apparently, this is where the medical billing shifts from an ER visit to "held for observation" patient visit—not because her medical condition had changed but because she was no longer considered by the medical billing code "in the ER."

Remember when Tammy was asked to be in the clinical research on snake venom upon arrival to her ER visit? This medical research required her permission for blood to be drawn independent of ER blood samples, in a repeated fashion and at scheduled intervals.

Tammy's blood had to be drawn over the first twenty-four-hour period. Those samples were drawn regularly and at increasingly greater time intervals. Following Tammy's discharge, she had returned to the ER the next day and then again about a week later to fulfill the requirements necessary for the medical study.

"We allowed ourselves to be lured into the belief that the doctor she was potentially assisting future snakebite victims and the medical community by remaining in the hospital to facilitate that process," Tammy said, looking back.

No hospital employee or healthcare professional explained to her or Dale that they would incur any potential billing ramifications tied to an extended stay or extra tests for the venomous-snake research.

Tammy's insurance coverage reverted from what she and Dale had understood was an emergency to an outpatient service. Without any warning, an additional 20 percent of all the hospital fees were automatically passed along to Tammy. From her and Dale's perspective, an outpatient service implied her needs were not critical and any emergency needs were over.

Had she and Dale been provided the benefit of this knowledge in advance and been advised that her continued care was no longer urgent, Tammy would have objected to the uncomfortable accommodations from the onset. Still, Tammy said that the hospital never bothered to follow up regarding her patient satisfaction with the services that she did receive.

Tammy will to this day still tell you in light of everything that transpired, the fees seemed excessive for the amount of service actually provided.

After spending only thirteen hours inside a hospital, she received one dosage of a drug, customary blood tests, and a tetanus shot. She was billed for fees amounting to almost $1,700, which is well in excess of the $300 emergency scenario.

Although she said her doctors seemed competent and caring, she and my brother-in-law felt duped. If this were not an emergency, then why was it a priority to collect this $300 while she was under duress?

To a millionaire, $1,700 may not seem like a lot of money, but for a middle-class family trying to make ends meet, it is a big chunk of their cash savings. It is a mortgage payment to most.

Tammy still feels everyone tied to this process apparently lacked the ability to understand how their decisions affected not only the patient's physical health but also his or her financial welfare.

Although the quality of care met Tammy and her husband's expectations, they are extremely frustrated with the lack of transparency that occurred regarding the costs.

Tammy also says it is difficult for her to imagine that these same services provided by a primary care physician during normal business hours would have been billed at these excessive rates.

When our dad heard about Tammy's experience, he laughed and said, "I guess that's the price you pay for allowing those doctors to practice their medicine on you. Ha! Ha! Ha! That's why they call their medical businesses medical 'practice,' because they're practicing medicine on you."

Crazy story, right?

Well, listen to this next one, about surgical instruments being "found" after surgeries were complete.

Did you know the chance of having a surgical instrument left inside your body after a surgery could be anywhere from 12.5 percent to 0.02 percent, depending on various statistics? According to Melanee Randall, a former operating room nurse at Boulder Community Health in Boulder, Colorado, this is true, and it happens more often than you might think.

Either way, the idea of having a foreign instrument left inside your body during a surgery is pretty creepy—especially when you consider the fact that an average of 250 instruments are used in any given surgery and that larger surgeries require an average of 600 tools. With all those moving parts, it is easy to see how these things could get misplaced on occasion.

This happened to my aunt Mary Lee in Alexandria, Louisiana, over twenty years ago.

Aunt Mary Lee was around 55 years old and needed to have surgery. No one really knew exactly what kind of surgery. We just knew it was somewhere on her abdomen, and you didn't question Aunt Mary Lee because she was considered to be the matriarch of our Louisiana family.

Mary Lee was my dad's older sister and one of the toughest women I knew. She had given birth to twelve children that lived and a set of twins that had died shortly after birth. She was strong physically, emotionally, mentally and spiritually. This woman was healthy as an ox and had the stamina to go to college in her forties to become a nurse. She made straight As while tending to her family's needs. Can you imagine going to school with twelve kids ages two to twenty-one?

Aunt Mary Lee headed off to surgery. My siblings and I, along with our parents, waited by the phone for the news of how it went.

The first report we got was that she did well, according to our uncle. The surgeon had just finished suturing her incision and then would be sending her to the recovery unit, he said.

Then we got another phone call. Apparently, while Aunt Mary Lee was in recovery, someone on the surgical staff in the OR had counted all the surgical tools used and realized, within minutes, one was missing.

My aunt was rushed back into the OR and an X-ray of the area they had operated on was quickly done. Lo and behold, they found the missing sponge still inside my aunt.

The surgeon was called back to remove the sponge, and my aunt recovered. After the news of what had happened got back to my aunt, she shrugged her shoulders and said, "These things happen sometimes. Thank God I'm okay." When most of our family heard this, they begged her to sue for malpractice, but she refused because she was a nurse and knew the doctor. She claimed this happened all the time.

Can you imagine if someone had not noticed the sponge was missing and my aunt had developed an infection? Gee whiz.

My other sister, Melody, explained that is why she and her family use boutique medicine—a growing cottage industry that serves the affluent.

Boutique medicine is when wealth tries to buy health—the caviar of healthcare or a health club of sorts. For a family of four, care cost would run about $60,000 annually in some medical-boutique practices.

In exchange, they get a full physical and wellness plan, 24-7 access to their doctor, wallet-sized CDs with their medical data recorded on it, and other services.

They also get a doctor with only 600 patients, compared to about 2,500 at a traditional practice. The boutique physician promises same-day or next-day appointments that last as long as the patient needs.

"Because of the nature of a smaller practice, it means I have more time to spend with patients and delve into problems," said Leonard Smith, a Florida-based boutique physician who is board certified in general, gastrointestinal, and vascular surgery. "I think one of the advantages of having fewer patients is that I have more time to appreciate those subtleties and nuances which can translate into big differences in terms of clinical decision-making and patient care."

"What that means is boutique medicine physicians have all the time necessary to provide complete access to their patients, extraordinary care and service, and home or office visits," Smith said. "We're able to offer total privacy because it's highly unlikely that we would ever have more than one patient at our office at any given time."

The offices do not have waiting rooms (or much waiting), and patients are encouraged to call Smith or his partners directly when they need to talk to a physician, Smith explained. If a patient needs to see a specialist, Smith will help find the best ones and even go to the appointment with them.

Annual fees for boutique medicine cover all doctor visits and any other services the office provides, such as X-rays, but outside treatment—an MRI, for example—would cost extra.

Many physicians call boutique practices "country-club medicine" and say it sends the wrong message.

"You still have this concept that you have to be a member of a club to get the healthcare you deserve," he said. "And that's just not true."

According to a physician who I will call Dr. H, as in HCP (healthcare provider), boutique physicians may come into his office once every other year.

"I'll have a lobby filled with patients, and the boutique physician will try to put me on the spot and ask me to give his or her patient an easy pass to skip ahead of my patients who have been waiting patiently for their turn," Dr. H said. "Medicine is not supposed to be about who will pay more money for better care.

"To me, the underlying issue is why physicians do this," Smith said. "And I think it's because physicians are just so frustrated and exasperated, particularly in primary care practices, by the amount of paperwork, the amount of hassle, and payment rates that don't reward for the services provided by primary care."

Smith is now retired.

Boutique medicine sounds great in theory, but when my brother-in-law's mother was diagnosed with colon cancer that progressed to her liver, he wanted her to see the doctor who was considered a guru with this disease. His brother had been trying for weeks to get her into Memorial Sloan Kettering, where the guru worked, to no avail.

I asked who they were trying to see. I was still working for the high-risk obstetrics company. A husband of one of the physicians who worked at Westchester Medical Center, Joe, had a connection to the guru. After explaining to Joe what was going on, I asked if he could help me get my aunt Zelda in to see her right away.

Joe asked me to give him a few minutes to make a call. Within ten minutes I got a call from Joe asking me how soon I could get Zelda to Sloan.

My point in sharing this story is to give you hope that it is not about the money; it is about connections with people you know and allowing them to help. But in order for people to help us, we have to ask. Right?

Throughout my professional life, I have come to believe that most people want to help, regardless of money. It's the insurance companies and government policies and regulations that cuff our hands, preventing us quick access to care.

Healthcare providers do not have the time they need to really be able to help you. Our culture has created a healthcare system that is smoke and mirrors. The tail wags the dog. And sadly, politicians know our country's healthcare system is too complicated to fix, even as many of them give lip service that they are hard at work on reforms.

Now, seven years after Obamacare was instituted, it's already falling apart.

If the government cannot fix it—who do you rely on? Just one word will suffice: yourself.

Chapter 6

My Own Healthcare Crisis

One freezing cold February morning in 2008, just before the sun was rising, I woke up tossing and turning. I remained still in bed, unable to gather enough energy to throw my legs over the side so my feet would somehow hit the floor, forcing my body to stand upright.

I decided to lie there a little longer. As I placed my cool hands on top of my face, I could also feel my head pounding. It felt as if someone were taking a screwdriver and using it with a hammer to tap into my skull.

My sheets were covered in blood. I had been bleeding vaginally off and on since October, but this morning was different than all the other times before. It was a morning like no other.

My sweet little English cocker spaniel, Beau, sensed my concern and was lying at the foot of the bed looking at me with his expressive furry face. He has a soft, cotton-like, chocolate and ivory curly coat, with cheese puff-colored marks above his eyebrows. He gingerly made his way up to my face, comforting me with a gentle kiss.

Beau's kiss somehow gave me the energy I needed to get out of bed. I then managed to make my way into the bathroom to shower, leaving a trail of blood behind. It was six degrees outside. The windows in the bathroom door were foggy from the shower's steam mixed with the cool air outside. There was three feet of snow. I wanted to walk Beau around the lake before I headed to the hospital.

Walking with Beau around the lake, being in nature, was how I started my daily meditation. Admiring the woods, deer, ducks, cows, and neighbors as they all walked by wishing me a wonderful day. About a mile from my house is the steepest hill on the lake.

As Beau and I started our climb, I began to notice my head and heart throbbing—throbbing so hard that I thought I might be having a heart attack. My vision began to blur. I felt dizzy. No one was in sight. I didn't know what was going on. All I knew was I needed to get home so I could call my friend who was a gynecologist.

Beau and I somehow managed to make it back. I do not even remember how, but we got home. I had snow on my knees. I thought I must have crawled after looking at myself in the mirror. All I could see was snow all over my pants. Blood was everywhere. I took another shower and dressed again.

I called a neighbor to take care of Beau as I headed off to work. I thought I could talk to my physician during lunch. Or should I say, I tried to drive to work. I made it about twenty miles and then had to turn around because my head was pounding harder and faster.

I called my best friend, who happens to be a doctor, and shared what was happening. She suggested I call my gynecologist and tell her how I was feeling. I was feeling so bad that I told Dr. Bravo I wanted to go to the ER.

Everyone who works in healthcare knows I hate being a patient. I would rather stick needles in my eye than be a patient. Maybe that is why I have a high pain threshold or tolerance.

Dr. Bravo suggested I come to her office first so she could fill out the paperwork to admit me to the hospital. She thought this would be faster and more comfortable for me. We knew we had to get in line for the operating room. It was going to be a while before my turn came.

While I was waiting, I started praying to my mother. Just as I sighed her name, I received a call from my uncle Sidney, her brother. They were like two peas in a pod. My sister and I had always looked up to our uncle. He had lived with us while he went to law school.

I shared with him what was going on. He then started chanting, "I think I can, I think I can," from the iconic children's book *The Little Engine That Could*. The moral of this story is understanding the value of optimism and hard work.

I smiled and felt comforted by his words because he and my mother used to read that story to me when I was a child.

It was now around 6:00 p.m. While waiting in the ER for the OR, I reflected on my healing journey. I had a similar health challenge involving my ovaries almost ten years before. It was shortly after I graduated from massage school. My classmate Mary had given me Caroline Myss's book called *Anatomy of the Spirit*, and my mother had given me Louise Hay's book called *You Can Heal Your Life*. The two authors' books were about how we create our own diseases within our minds, which then show up in our bodies.

The ovaries in Hay's book represent the point of creation and creativity; and in Myss' book, she talks about the imbalance in primarily romantic relationships. Mine had definitely been imbalanced, then and now.

I was asking myself why I had not learned this lesson. Why was it showing up in my body again? But this time more serious. I had been diagnosed a few days prior with a myoma on my cervix. My physician and I had talked about several options. One was to wait a few days or so and give it a chance to drop farther down my uterus—very much like how a baby's head drops before delivery—so she could do an ablation. A laser thermal ablation is the surgical removal of body tissue by a laser beam.

However, I was bleeding much more heavily now, so much so that my hematocrit level was at six. Normally it is twelve, which meant I had lost half of my body's blood volume. This explained why I had such a pounding headache, was so dizzy, and why my heart was pounding like it was outside my body. I looked whiter than a ghost.

As I type this last sentence, I can hear the Indigo Girls singing "Galileo." While waiting for my epidural, I couldn't help but ask myself how long was it going to take my soul to get it right.

As I was being transferred into the OR, I was being told by Dr. Bravo that my condition was more serious than she had thought. She and my maternal-fetal medicine (MFM) specialist friend were afraid I was bleeding out and did not want to play around. They were now suggesting a partial hysterectomy—removing my bassinet (uterus) and leaving my rattles (ovaries). So I had successfully healed my ovaries from ten years ago.

When I heard the word *hysterectomy*, I began to freak out. Not that I wanted to have any kids, especially at forty-six years old, but I knew from the books I had read that this was my center of creativity. I was an artist and relied on my creativity in sales as well as to make a living.

I no longer felt like I was giving a natural-delivery birth to my childlike growth as Dr. Bravo had described earlier. I was now being whisked away for an emergency—having a cesarean section to remove this thing.

Upon discharge from the hospital, Dr. Bravo told me I would probably be off from work until the end of April because my iron was so low from my blood loss. She was concerned that having low iron levels could cause me to faint or pass out. My job required me to drive a lot, and she did not want me to become a hazard to myself or anyone else.

Two months off from work, feeling low, and in the dead of winter. What would I do during this time?

As the saying goes: We plan. God laughs.

And little did I know, this would be when my spiritual journey would begin to kick into high gear.

My girlfriend Alexandra Harris, from back home in Gainesville, invited me to her Outrageous Outcomes workshop.

"Outrageous Outcomes," the name I helped her create years ago to describe her personal-growth workshop. The activities she uses to help her participants heal are far from normal.

"I want to help you tap into the understanding that the power within you is greater than any barrier in your body or outside of you," Alexandra explained to me.

The workshop included numerous physical challenges: glass walking, snapping and breaking an arrow with our throats, bending a metal rebar while two people hold it up together with each person's throat, and lastly, walking unharmed across a twelve-foot runway of 1,800-degree hot coals (better known as fire walking).

I know what you are thinking. The world does not need more people who can walk on fire. We need people who are willing to embrace healing. Well, for some, that may look like walking across the fire. The firewalk symbolizes our ability to break limiting beliefs that we all carry inside of us—beliefs that may be restricting us or may be causing disease in our bodies.

I was mesmerized by Alexandra starting her workshop by saying she was going to explore some simple truths. There are only three primary colors in existence—red, blue, and yellow—but look what Michelangelo did with those three colors, she shared.

There are only twelve notes—but look what Chopin, Beethoven, and Vivaldi did with those twelve notes, she continued.

There are twenty-six letters in the alphabet—but look what Jefferson, Franklin, Walt Whitman, and Shakespeare did with those letters. And there are only ten digits—but look what von Braun and Einstein did with those ten digits.

Now I was beginning to get it.

These realizations spoke to me more than the firewalk itself because they encouraged thinking beyond the ordinary limitations of these examples.

Had these artists and scientists she mentioned stopped at these simple truths, they would not have created their masterpieces, which not only changed their perceptions but also made our world better!

I now believe that this is the way we need to start thinking about our own healthcare.

This experience was just the beginning of my spiritual awakening, and it inspired me to take more control of my life, creating my own healthcare team outside the hospital and traditional doctor's office.

I changed my mind-set entirely. I began my own study— exploring unconventional healers and other options, such as a healthier diet, motion therapy (exercise program), a spiritual practice such as ACIM, and spending more time with like-minded people.

Perhaps the most beautiful lesson and the greatest gift

that the walk gave me was having the courage and confidence in life to do something to overcome any barrier—between us, our health, and any goal we are pursuing.

What I learned was this. We cannot, in our minds, figure out how to get across this barrier known as the firewalk. Standing in front of this extremely hot fire, underneath a canopy of stars, feeling the dirt between my toes, while bugs crawled over the top of my feet. I had to wait until I was guided to walk by my internal voice.

It was like the universe was paving my way.

After the initial step in introducing me to the fire's path, I gracefully and slowly relished my adventure across the coals. I could hear coals crunching, but no attention or thoughts from my mind interrupted my trip. Not once did I think about being burned.

A few days later, I returned to New York. I got a phone call from my friend Kathy, who has her DNP in nursing. She suggested I go to an energy healer. Kathy lives in Bayside, Queens, which is about two hours south of where I live. She thought I had a lot of stuck energy that was keeping me, well, stuck.

Kathy shared with me the name and phone number of an energy healer near my home. Her name is Jeanett Dauffau. Jeanett was one of the first registered nurses to get a degree in natural medicine. Her office is in Olive Branch, New York, near Woodstock.

I always looked forward to my sessions with Jeanett. We started off by sharing what was happening in my world since our last visit. Then she would pull out her animal deck of cards. Each card had a beautiful environmental portrait of an animal in its natural surroundings. The animal on the card represented a story of their superpowers.

I would draw four cards from the deck, and Jeanett would apply each to my life in the past, present, and future. She would then ask me to move to her bodywork table, and she would use oils to balance my energy—my life force.

One day, after doing the cards and before she had me get on the table, she handed me an aluminum tennis racket. She then placed a bunch of pillows on top of the table and asked me to breathe deeply in and out. After a few minutes, she directed me to hit the pillows with the racket as hard as I could.

I took a few swings and said, "So, what am I supposed to do now?" She shrugged her shoulders and then asked me how I felt, and she said, "Keep swinging!"

I swung a few more times and said I did not get it. She then shared with me that she felt I had buried a lot of anger in my body, causing an unhealthy imbalance that she could feel stuck in my aura.

Next thing you know, I took a few deep breaths as I felt my body temperature start to heat up. I began to swing harder and harder. She then asked me to put words to my feelings and asked me who was I angry with. I said my dad. She then coached me on swinging more. Before you knew it, I broke the aluminum tennis racket.

I then started laughing and said, "I guess you were right. I was angry! Ha ha ha!"

Jeanett then asked me to take a look in the mirror. I looked at least ten years younger and felt lighter.

Driving back home, I was admiring the beautiful country-side of the Hudson Valley as I crossed the Rhinebeck/Kingston Bridge on Route 199. I learned there is definitely truth in the body, mind, and spirit connections. And sometimes you have to keep going back to the past to heal emotional wounds that never healed enough to develop a scar.

Here is where this lesson I had to learn starts to creep back into my life now. Once again, I am questioning our healthcare system and how it glosses over the connection between our emotional and physical health. It's designed to treat the sick physical symptoms—but never explore the mental avenues that might have led to the illness itself.

My friend and mentor Marianne Williamson, author of *Return to Love* (based on ACIM), says we really do not have a healthcare system. It's really a sickness-care system.

ACIM states in lesson 136 that sickness is a defense against the truth. No one can heal unless we understand what purpose sickness seems to serve.

Sickness is not an accident. And now, after many years of reflection and seeing the system up close, I know that this is true.

Chapter 7

My Plan: Healing Begins with Our Spirits

It was the last Wednesday in June—hump day. I was quickly reminded I work on the front line of the frustration healthcare professionals are feeling, whether they work in a hospital, a wound-care center, a doctor's office or a clinic.

I was parked, sitting in my car just outside of a doctor's office. I was there to follow up on a few patients whose negative-pressure wound-therapy (NPWTP) devices from my company were still pending because of information that was missing. The insurance company would not approve the request until they received the necessary information from the physician who had ordered the device as a part of their patient's treatment.

While on my cell phone with the customer service representative at our home office, my district manager texted me to call him.

He shared with me that a nurse in one of my wound-care centers had complaints about me. It struck me as odd since I had not had an in-person conversation or in-service session with her in over a year and a half.

I remembered in August 2015 talking with this particular nurse after she had requested someone from our company conduct in-service training for the nurses in her hospital. She had wanted someone to come in at 11:00 p.m. to teach her staff how to do dressing changes. I had explained to her that I didn't cover the hospital and had given her the phone number of someone who could help her.

Several months had passed. Our company had received an NPWT referral from her for one of her patients. The wound measurements were missing. Her patient's insurance company would not approve the NPWT without them. I had called her phone number at her wound care center. Her colleague had answered the phone. Before I could identify myself and state the reason for my call, her colleague had screamed in my ear, "She's with a patient."

I had then replied, "That's why I'm calling. It's about her patient, for whom she has referred NPWT." I had explained to her colleague that this RN had forgotten to include the wound measurements in her request, and the patient's insurance company would not approve NPWT without those measurements.

About an hour later, I had gotten a call from the program director at the wound-care center saying I had been rude. Confused and at a loss for words, I had apologized and then explained why I had called.

After I had hung up with the program director, I had shaken it off and chalked this incident up to how busy our healthcare professionals are, along with their frustrations with insurance companies continually creating more paperwork, in turn delaying their treatment plan for a patient.

By then, I was thinking about spiritual laws and karma. I thought to myself that I'd hate to be this nurse, knowing the karma she was creating by trying to get me in trouble for doing my job.

Just like her and all other healthcare professionals, I am here for the patient too.

This ugly incident left me counting the days to Friday night and to my weekend retreat with Marianne Williamson, called Miraculous Mind, Miraculous Life. My girlfriends Alexandra and Kristi were coming to join me.

Several months before I had signed up for this retreat, I had been ambivalent as to whether or not I wanted to participate. Then I had been reminded by Marianne that it was my idea for her to do a weekend retreat at Omega Institute. The Omega Institute is located near where I live. Typically, on most weeks, I drive an hour and a half each Tuesday evening from my home to the city (New York City) for Marianne's "A Course in Miracles" lectures. They mean so much to me and are always worth the extra time and travel.

During our retreat, a woman who was in remission from stage III cancer asked Marianne about healing spiritually from a physical illness. I learned from Marianne's answer that the source of sickness is lovelessness, but it may not be lovelessness on the part of the person who has contracted the illness. When you look at how many carcinogens there are in our foods, air, and grounds, it's easy to conclude that we make money more important than love. We talk about deregulation like it's some higher good, said Williamson.

Deregulation means you don't have to protect our environment. The EPA is taking scientists off its main panels. Dow Chemicals is allowed to sell pesticides that all the scientists said should be banned permanently because of carcinogens.

This insanity is a part of our whole society. We acquiesce to something like this and then tell ourselves it's OK because in allowing deregulation, we've made it easier for businesses to create more jobs.

I loved how, during the retreat, Marianne explained that

we were all going to take a train out of here—meaning life. It's just that some of us would be taking the 10:05 train, and others the 5:15 train.

I think the lesson here in preserving our health is to always look at our part of contracting the sickness. We need to deepen our thinking in this arena by seeing a mind, body, and spirit connection.

Such understanding, however, is a lifetime process or journey. Getting there and coming around to this mind-set doesn't happen overnight.

I can remember first being introduced to "A Course in Miracles" (ACIM) in the late eighties, when a friend gave me the book, *A Woman's Worth*. When my mother saw me reading this book, she took it upon herself to hand me the book *Return to Love.* My mother—well on her own journey—told me that if I liked the book I was reading, I would love this one.

Both were written by Marianne. And in hindsight, she was already preaching great truth. I just didn't understand it fully then.

Fast-forward to five years later: I was in an imbalanced relationship and having health issues with my ovaries.

After I resolved that relationship, I moved to New York, where I would meet Marianne for the first time at one of her ACIM lectures that she gave after the 9/11 attacks. I was still trying to listen, but I still hadn't fully learned the lesson.

Fast-forward again.

Seven years later, I was in another imbalanced relationship and contracted a myoma.

Along the way, over those years, I had tried to improve. I had made better choices with food, exercise, yoga, and a few other things. But for some reason, I hadn't fully integrated my new beliefs about myself. And I hadn't healed my old beliefs that may have kept me stuck, attracting illness to my body.

After our weekend retreat was over, my friends and I headed back to our homes—back to the "real" world, the place where we would get to practice what we just learned.

Starting our day with prayer and meditations. Plugging/connecting our bodies to God—our source of the divine light—whom we learned works much like a lamp you plug into a socket in your house. Such action creates electricity to light up your room.

Today, as I write, it's July 4, 2017, America's 421st birthday. According to Gregg Braden, our bodies are made to live nine hundred years. "It's the first hundred years that are the most challenging."

I was born in 1961. The first year in office for John Fitzgerald "Jack" Kennedy, better known as JFK, our thirty-fifth president and one of our most admired. Although I was only a couple of months old when he made this statement, it is one of my favorite political quotes: "And so, my fellow Americans, ask not what your country can do for you, ask what you can do for your country."

During my meditation today, I finally understood what I call the medical remedy for our political healthcare system issues. It's simple and could solve a lot of problems immediately.

I call it "the two-cents solution," or the Two-Cents Federal Sales Tax Healthcare Bill. I say "two cents" because I care about and value you and your two cents.

My healthcare solution would eliminate insurance companies and the hassles for healthcare providers while providing us with better healthcare and erasing high healthcare premiums.

Insurance companies can focus on other markets such as liability, home, rental, and car insurance.

Imagine if "we the People of the United States" demanded that our politicians create a "two-cent bill." We could afford Medicare for all. That is right, you heard me—by earmarking two cents of every dollar spent on nonessential goods and services in the United States toward our healthcare costs, we would be able to cover everyone in the United States' medical bills.

Keep in mind we are already taxed on essential and nonessential goods and services.

I got this idea from the old math question that someone asked me when I was in the third grade. I learned the power of a penny. The penny also carries a note on its front: In God we trust.

If you had the choice of my giving you a million dollars right now or the sum of a penny doubled every day for thirty days, which would you choose? Most people might quickly respond with a million dollars, of course, before doing any math.

Not so fast. For some people like myself, with my similar intuition (the guidance from my inner voice), we would choose the sum of a penny doubled every day for thirty days.

I'll show you why you'd want the sum of a penny a day doubled for thirty days. It equals $10.7 million.

After taking out my calculator and checking my math, I googled my question, and sure enough, Bloomberg's Adam Johnson, on his program called *Chart Attack*, asked CEO Chuck Akre, "Does a penny doubled every day for thirty days equal $10.7 million?"

Akre confirmed that the formula was very true. Akre said it was a simple lesson in compounded return.

Akre also said most people aren't comfortable doing the math.

Compounding returns? I thought to myself in this moment, Isn't this what our insurance companies are doing with the money we pay them for our health insurance policies?

However, once we pay them, they have the right to change the original policy we signed with them within days. All they are required by our government to do is to publish this change to our personal policies on their websites. Insurance companies do not have to send you a letter informing you of any changes, either.

Talk about anti-consumer.

Guess how many people in our country don't own a computer or better yet know how to use one? My father is eighty-three years old and doesn't own a computer, nor would he know how to use a computer to go to his insurance company's website.

Even if my father knew how to use a computer to go to his health insurance company to find the changes in his policy, he would be angered because this was not the insurance policy he signed or bought. He would call it a breach of contract—a bait and switch.

Our insurance companies are hoping we're not doing the math. They are hoping we never question or create a revolution against their higher-math games.

Our insurance policies are rather like us going to the Kentucky Derby horse race and placing a bet on a horse to win a profit. We're given a ticket upon the bet placed. It's very similar to when we give money to an insurance company for a healthcare policy.

At the Kentucky Derby, we place a two-dollar bet without even questioning if and how we're going to get paid. We understand the risk and the gains. Just like the insurance company knows its risk and gains when it gives us a health-care policy.

When betting at the Kentucky Derby on a chance for our horse to win, the ticket represents our contract. This, too, is very similar to how our insurance company is betting on the chance to win—with the expiration date on each of our health insurance policies. The insurance company is betting on us not needing healthcare while it rakes in the profits.

The biggest difference between the Kentucky Derby and our health insurance companies is, at the Kentucky Derby, there are no profits if your horse loses. Insurance companies get paid on our insurance premiums regardless if we use our healthcare policy or not.

The other difference between insurance companies and horse racing is that with the insurance company, yearly "race" profits involve a large pool of policyholders, not just one horse. You can place a bet on more than one horse, but each bet costs more money. Right?

Do you see where I'm going here? Every year is a new race for insurance companies with higher profits and less care provided to you and me—the very folks who pay for these policies in the first place.

Please don't get lost in the hope that our government will fix this insurance race for us. Our government is one of the sponsors for this healthcare insurance company race, just like the Kroger Company, Yum!, Sentient Jet, and Stella Artois are to the Kentucky Derby.

Realize, too, that it is not in our politicians' best interests to have a one-payer healthcare system—even if some lawmakers continue to give such a notion lip service.

Perhaps if our original Founding Fathers were in office, this would have never happened. Why do you think the abolitionists or the women's suffragettes or Rev. Martin Luther King Jr. took to the streets and marched?

They stood up to our politicians because they were not being heard by them. And they followed their own individual moral compasses within. Meanwhile, these lawmakers, whose health insurance is a perk of their elected jobs, listened with their greed instead of their hearts—even for their fellow men and women who elected them.

Let's go back to the math for a second.

According to Worldometers, the current population of the United States is 326,496,823. We comprise 4.3 percent of the world's population. In February 2014, *Forbes* magazine reported US healthcare spending was over $3.8 trillion.

If we take two cents (.02) and multiply it by 326,496,823, we get 652,993,646. We need four hundred trillion pennies to equal $4 trillion, which is more than the what we spent in America on healthcare in 2014.

Now multiply this by all the nonessential consumer goods and services categories in America.

For instance, let's look at these six nonessential goods and services categories we could tax: fast food and potato chips (not including fine dining), transportation (Highway Trust Fund), aircraft, recreational boating, tobacco, and alcohol.

Potatogrower.com reported that in 2015, US consumers spent $7.5 billion on potato chips—an average of roughly $23 for every man, woman, and child, according to Packaged Facts, a market research publisher.

If that blows your mind, let's look at fast food. Fast food revenues hit $200 billion in 2015, a bewildering increase from the $6 billion reported in revenues in 1970, according to an industry analysis by FranchiseHelp.com. That equates to about $625 per person in the country spent at fast food restaurants for the year.

So, let's make this more fun. How many Big Macs do you think Americans consume on average in a year?

McDonald's estimates that it sells about 550 million Big Macs each year in the United States. That breaks down to one every seventeen seconds.

Let's look at highways and transportation. Did you know the United States has a Highway Trust Fund?

The Highway Trust Fund is a transportation fund in the United States which generates money from a federal fuel tax of 18.4 cents per gallon on gasoline, and 24.4 cents per gallon on diesel fuel and related excise taxes. Currently, it has two accounts: the Highway Account which funds road construction and other surface transportation projects, and a smaller Mass Transit Account which supports mass transit.

According to Wikipedia, at the end of the 2015 fiscal year, this federal excise tax raised $98.3 billion, or 3 percent of total federal tax revenue.

This Fund finances most federal government spending on highways and mass transit. Revenues for the trust fund come from transportation-related excise taxes, primarily federal taxes on gasoline and diesel fuel.

Recently, however, the trust fund has needed significant transfers of general revenues to remain solvent, according to the tax policy center.

Fuel is to transportation as healthcare is to our bodies. Why is it acceptable for our country to support a tax on transportation to maintain this system, but not a tax to maintain healthcare?

Now let's look at how much Americans spent on aircrafts and boats in 2013.

According to *Forbes*, in 2013 the United States spent $150 billion. Yes, that's just on flying, regardless of if it is business or not.

And for water babies, according to the National Marine Manufacturers Association, Americans spent $121 billion in 2013 on recreational boating.

So now, you're probably wondering how much Americans spend on tobacco and alcohol. Well, according to the Centers for Disease and Control and Prevention, during 2016 $258 billion in cigarettes were sold in the United States. If we include cigars, add another $12 billion in sales. Are you also wanting to know about marijuana sales? According to a January 2017 HuffPost article, Americans and Canadians spent $53.3 billion on marijuana in 2016.

Surprising—according to *Fortune's* online article in 2016, the volume of liquor was only $25.2 billion. The United States beer market, according to Nielsen's website, was more than $37 billion in 2017. On September 27, 2017, Emma Balter of *Wine Spectator* reported that Americans would spend $219.9 billion on wine.

See where I'm going with this idea of a nonessential consumer tax? And these are only five areas.

In 2015, the Bureau of Labor Statistics' annual Consumer Expenditure Survey found that the average American spends $140 a day on essential goods—essential goods meaning food and shelter.

Steve Kattell, owner and manager of Kattell and company, a certified public accounting firm providing services exclusively to not-for-profit organizations, was intrigued with my solution and did the math for us.

So, $140 per US citizen per day times 2 percent equals $2.80; $2.80 times 326,496,823 US citizens equals $914,191,104 sales tax collections nationally per day.

Finally, $914,191,104 times 365 equals $333,679,753,106— that's only 9 percent of the $3.8 trillion needed.

Kattell said doing the math backward, it looks like you need a sales tax of 23 percent: $3.8 trillion divided by 365 divided by 326,496,823 equals $32 per citizen per day. That means we would need a sales tax of approximately 23 percent more on essential services and nonessential goods and services to get the $3.8 trillion needed ($32/$140 = 22.78%). This means an additional $32 per person per day to make my two-cent federal sales tax work.

After reviewing how much Americans spend on driving, smoking, drinking, flying, and recreational boating, it is easier to see how quickly two cents per dollar add up fast. And these are only six categories.

So my question is, why not consider my idea for a two-cent federal sales tax?

My healthcare resolution would include tourists, illegal residents, or green card holders. If something were to happen to them while in the United States, they would be covered because they spent money here.

Currently, .05 percent of sales tax collection goes to health and welfare.

My point is, if we created a national healthcare tax such as the two-cent federal sales tax that I am proposing, we would not need insurance companies. We would create a one-payer system and have plenty of money to take care of anyone who is in our country without anyone having to pay.

At the end of our tax year, if you or a company wanted to pay more money for our healthcare system, you could. For your generous donation or contribution toward a healthier

America, you could be rewarded a dollar-for-dollar tax credit and write-off.

Anyone who spent money outside of our two-cents healthcare tax on a nontraditional healing modality that was not approved by the FDA would also get a dollar-for-dollar tax credit as long as he or she had a receipt of record for the amount rendered until cleared by the FDA. This would honor folks who practice healthier choices in their daily lifestyles, embracing the body, mind, and spirit connection that I believe is crucial to wellness.

Our current system is not working because only 53 percent of Americans pay income tax, where a large percentage of healthcare costs are paid.

Chris Murphy, a Democratic senator from Connecticut, made a video that appeared on Now This.

This is what he claims (in my transcripts from his video)— much of which is inaccurate if not downright false. But it is a narrative created by the left to explain why the Obama plan continues to fail.

Murphy noted:

Obamacare isn't failing. Trump is sabotaging it. With all the attention on the House health-care-repeal bill that steals healthcare from millions of Americans and jacks cost up for everybody else, I want to make sure that you know that the president of the United States is, right now as we speak, trying to sabotage the American Healthcare System as a political retribution against people that wouldn't work with him. Here's what President Trump is doing: he's trying to ruin the American healthcare system to create a crisis that then will necessitate this piece of legislation. It all started when he issued an executive order.

Murphy continued:

An executive order that commands all federal agencies to start undermining the Affordable Care Act and his agencies listened. The IRS decided to stop enforcing the individual mandate that was the underpinning of the Affordable Care Act. That has resulted in insurance companies all across the country jacking their rates up, explicitly because they don't believe that healthy people will buy insurance. It continued when the Trump administration stopped funding the advertising of the Affordable Care Act and the health care exchanges. When President Trump was sworn into office, open enrollment was happening, and we were on a pace to set records, but when President Trump started talking down the Affordable Care Act and pulled the advertising for it, people stopped signing up and we ended up having somewhere around three hundred thousand to five hundred thousand people who didn't sign up for the Affordable Care Act because Trump pulled the advertising and now HHS [Health and Human Services] is threatening to pull the subsidies that go to insurance companies to incentivize them to take part in these markets. They've just committed to sending the subsidies on a month-by-month basis, which has left every insurance company in the country with the potential decision to pull out of the marketplaces without the assurance that these subsidies are going to continue.

Murphy added:

So, there is a very purposeful, intentional, planned strategy that this administration is undertaking to try to weaken and sabotage the US healthcare system so that they can have a reason for why this repeal bill has to pass, despite the fact it will result in millions of people losing coverage, rates going up, and benefits going down. You need to know about this campaign of

sabotage so you can speak up about it. I say let's take to
the streets like our ancestors before us and march so our
voices can be heard! Why, heck, look at the abolitionists,
women's suffragettes, Martin Luther King Jr., and now
Sister Giant.

Sister Giant is a movement on the intersection of consciousness and politics. If our votes are not representing our voices ("we the People of the United States") need to take action so our voices can be heard by our politicians.

I am joining this fight. I may not agree with everything the Obama administration did, but I do agree we need a single-payer system in this country.

Ask any physician or healthcare professional what the solution is and they will agree to a single-payer system because it is the insurance companies tying their hands, preventing them from ordering the appropriate tests upon request in order to diagnose people sooner than later. In healthcare, we will all agree, in most cases, the sooner the diagnosis, the sooner the treatment, the better the outcome.

Insurance companies are keeping you and me from the quality care we each need and are also keeping the healthcare providers from doing their jobs.

In Marianne Williamson's Sister Giant movement video, posted on YouTube, she argues that the time is now for a rising-up as people speak out and push back against corporate profiteering that is imperiling society.

She notes:

Our government has been sewn into this straitjacket. It
functions now at the behest of a corporate aristocracy,
bought and sold to the highest bidder: oil companies,

pharmaceutical companies, chemical companies, big agriculture, defense contractors, financial institutions. First, they get what they want, and then whatever crumbs that fall from the table of power after they've feasted are divvied up among the people.

Well, some very bad ideas have produced some very bad results from this already. From climate change to the poisoning of our food supply to raging terrorism to unsustainable inequality to the dismantling of our democracy itself. And all that will continue until we change the trajectory of things in a big way. When money rules our government the way it does now, creating an insane political establishment and sociopathic economy, it's time for a democratic revolution in America, a revolution of light and consciousness and love.

We need to read. We need to think. We need to organize. We need to march. We need to meditate. We need to support the right candidates. We need to be the right candidates. We need to vote. We need to be noisy. We need to be unapologetic. We need to be willing to be dismissed. We need to be awake and alive and full of love and telling truths to power. And If we do, and when we do, then America will break out of this ridiculous corporate straitjacket that imperils us the way it does now.

Our government is being held captive and only we, the people, the citizens of this country, can free it—which is fine because we can do that. For we have a power inside us more powerful than all the powers of the world.

To wit: if our healthcare system is to change, we must consider a huge rage against this machine.

Chapter 8

As Long as You Have Money

I am a journalist, a fact finder, a truth seeker by trade. And those skills stick with me when I have questions. I like to do my research. And when I have more questions, I meditate and pray.

This issue of why we simply cannot do a better job providing health insurance for all of us really got under my skin. I could not stop thinking about it, so I started surfing the internet in search of when insurance companies began. I asked God to show me why our current healthcare system does not work.

Did you know that before 1973 it was illegal in the United States to profit off of healthcare? The Health Maintenance Organization Act of 1973 passed by Nixon changed everything.

As I prayed and quieted myself to listen, I received an answer to my question. And it was not pretty. Our US politicians are in bed with the insurance companies and have been for decades, making it tough to adopt a single-payer system without creating a medical revolution.

But that is what it would take for real change to occur—a revolution.

From all of my experience in healthcare as a medical sales representative and as a patient, I have come to believe that a single-payer system is our answer. Bernie Sanders was actually running on a single-payer healthcare system in 2016 against President Trump and former first lady Hillary Clinton. His idea resonated with a lot of people but also got caught in the political fray. I think it is a notion worth revisiting in earnest.

Sanders, who has suggested a new plan, wants to continue the collection of money the way we do now—where we pay out of several funds—sales tax, property tax, employer tax, FICA, plus an additional increase in the inheritance tax and capital gains tax. I am suggesting a true single-payer with one tax—a single consumption tax.

Perhaps my ancestors before me were chiming in during my meditation, talking to me from afar. They saw this corruption firsthand.

My maternal great-grandfather served in the Florida House of Representatives in 1929. In 1963, his son and my great-uncle Etter Thomas Usher served in the Florida Senate for four years, representing the Twenty-First District, which included Dixie, Gilchrist, and Levy Counties. Uncle Etter, my mother's namesake, was proud to be known as a porkchopper.

When Uncle Etter was asked if he would run for a second term, he graciously passed, saying he could do more good on the outside as a farmer and a cattleman than he could do on the inside as a state senator.

Uncle Etter shared with me many times throughout my childhood and adult years how corrupt our government was then. Keep in mind, he served from 1963 to 1967, fifty years ago. A pretty powerful statement, right? And yet all it took was one term as a state lawmaker to show him how deep corruption's tentacles really went. The system was fixed. He saw it up close.

Looking back on my family members who served in our

Florida State Senate, both Republican and Democrat, I think our family's most talked-about politician was my second cousin Charles D. Williams. Charles was a Republican Party Florida state senator from 1992 to 1996 who served only one term because in his preelection for his second term, he announced he was in favor of initiating tort reform. We called Charles "Uncle" because he was Mom's first cousin and closer to her age.

Before Uncle Charles went into politics, he had a career in insurance.

Uncle Charles was pushed out of office by trial attorneys because he wanted tort reform for Florida. Tort reform would cap the amount of money an attorney could make off of a malpractice case. High-dollar attorneys did not like that because it took away their power, so he had to go!

I feel sure my own father and yes, my uncle, will think I am going crazy or, better yet, trying to get myself arrested by telling you, my reader and fellow American, what I have found. But in writing this book, I can no longer stay silent. It is my civic duty and moral compass directing me to share the truth about our healthcare system, which is hurting us all and frankly destined to fail.

But before I share with you the truth about who benefits more from our current system, I would like to ask you to ponder your own experience. Have you been asked recently by a physician or physician's office who your insurer is, meaning who is the healthcare insurance company your medical benefits are covered by? Now, that's typically the first question you get, and woe to those who have none.

Let's take a step back to a personal experience. My friend, Carmela's son, was diagnosed with acute lymphocytic leukemia at twenty-one months old in 1980. Carmela remembers back when insurance covered everything. Carmela's son was known as the "miracle baby" because the chances of the treatment given by his physicians were slim for a remission.

Her son achieved a remission. However, almost thirty-seven years later, Carmela had noticed her son's jaw "not looking right." Carmela quickly called her doctor and made an appointment for her son to be seen.

Her family physician ran a series of tests and learned that her son had cancer in his jaw. Carmela's son received radiation and once again went into remission.

For almost thirty-seven years after her son's last episode, life for Carmela and him seemed pretty great until her son began to have seizures.

Carmela's son was diagnosed with a meningioma, a tumor that is usually benign, arising from the meningeal tissue of the brain. Her son's physicians thought it could have been caused by the radiation given to his jaw years before.

Camela's son's physician operated to remove these tumors.

Fast-forward to April 2017. Nearly thirty-seven years after her son's tumors were removed, he began to have seizures again.

Once again, Carmela called her son's physicians to make an appointment. His physician wanted him to have an MRI.

Carmela called the MRI center to make an appointment. They asked Carmela for her son's insurance and then promised to call her back in a few minutes to make an appointment. Carmela was anxious because she feared she was losing time. She had been here before and knew that the quicker her physician could get the MRI results, the sooner he could make a diagnosis and the sooner her son could start treatment. Carmela also knew from all the times before with her son, the sooner the treatment, the better the outcome—meaning his survival rate.

An hour later, Carmela's phone rang. It was the MRI center. They could get her son in by the next week, but apparently, they did not accept his insurance. The MRI cost several thousands of dollars.

Carmela quickly found another MRI center who would take her son's insurance as well. But she also learned that it would be eight weeks before her son could have his MRI done.

By now, Carmela was frightened and feeling hopeless. She knew time was running out for her son to have a good prognosis without the MRI. She grabbed her cell phone and called the first MRI center back and asked if they could still do her son's MRI the next week if she paid cash. Within seconds, Carmela and her son were given an appointment.

My point in sharing Carmela and her son's story is to illustrate how cash rules. I also want to show you how insurance companies are delaying care needed for good outcomes. Had she not had $2,000, her son would have waited two months before having his MRI. And this could have truly made his problem worse.

Within two months, he was diagnosed with four new tumors. The biggest tumor, which was causing his seizures, was removed within a month after the MRI results were reviewed.

Insurance companies are delaying care to save money and increase their profits, especially for their CEOs and our politicians.

Our healthcare system today is set up to grease the pockets of our lawmakers, of big pharma, massive healthcare corporations, and insurances companies, many of which seek to delay and dismiss any alternative therapy as valid.

In the eighties, Carmela's health insurance gave her pretty much the green light without a co-pay when physicians ordered tests or procedures, but not today. Much has changed with our health insurance policies. We are paying more in return for less medical treatment, and our physicians' hands are tied. They cannot treat us without tests being done for their diagnosis to be made.

It is not that the physicians do not care; it is that insurance companies are not allowing proper tests to be done in a timely manner. Insurance companies are purposefully creating more work for our physicians and staff to do in order to receive payment. You need only read through the Affordable Care Act as it is now written to see its onerous burdens on doctors, which add to their costs as well as the time they can see and treat their patients.

One day, as I was thinking about our failing system, I remembered Bellevue Hospital is the first public hospital in the United States. Bellevue served everyone from presidents to paupers. This institution was founded in 1736 as an almshouse, a six-bed ward of last resort. It is still open after 280 years. When it started caring for patients, there was no such thing as health insurance. So births, surgeries, and enduring illnesses were in most cases taken care of at home. People then simply went to places like Bellevue to die. It appears as if we are coming full circle, with folks going into hospitals to die because it is too expensive to hire healthcare professionals to take care of them in their home. And most insurances do not cover home care for folks to die in their own homes.

I fear that is the new direction we are headed.

Our current trajectory, with insurance denying treatment because of money, refusing to cover needed equipment and pay for tests—the rising costs of it all may force us back into our homes for healthcare with hospitals becoming places only to die.

I also wonder about the young folks who may have a dream to become doctors, like I once did.

I am pretty sure most who are drawn to a career in medicine do not realize, at least not in the beginning, that nowadays, when they open their offices, they have a six-hundred-pound gorilla sitting in the room alongside their patients: government and corporate greed. But that is the reality.

I hope medical schools explain this to students—that their wide-eyed students who hoped to heal are entering a business now, not a calling. The system is no longer set up to heal people. It is set up to make money and to ration or deny care to those who cannot afford it.

Chapter 9
Way Beyond Politics

While many in our divided nation have sought to lay the healthcare problems at the feet of a political party, I feel it is right to say this: please do not get caught up in the Republican or Democratic party debate. I believe our political culture wants us to argue with one another as a distraction from what is really going on.

All you have to do is look at the records to see that both Republican and Democrat politicians are being paid.

Influence peddling is real, and it works. Both sides have their hands out. That is a fact.

Let us take a hard look at the money trail. Where is our money going when we pay our healthcare premiums for our healthcare policies?

According to OpenSecrets.org, a website created by the Center for Responsive Politics (OSOCFRP), in the 2016 presidential election, total contributions to Democrats and Republicans were $85,209,938.

Who gave them the most money? From 2015 to 2016, the top twenty companies that contributed to Democrats, Republicans, liberal groups, and conservatives were as follows:

1.   Starr Companies – $15,266,251

2.   Blue Cross / Blue Shield – $6,606,407

3. New York Life Insurance – $2,816,858

4. National Association of Insurance & Financial Advisors – $2,212,450

5. Cooperative of American Physicians – $1,957,046

6. AFLAC Inc – $1,933,323

7. Council of Insurance Agents & Brokers – $1,676,329

8. MetLife Inc. – $1,632,944

9. Independent Insurance Agents & Brokers of America: This is wrongIndependent Insurance Agents & Brokers of America – $1,611,475

10. USAA – $1,593,309

11. Massachusetts Mutual Life Insurance – $1,470,511

12. Prudential Financial – $1,394,802

13. Nationwide – $1,374,761

14. Northwestern Mutual – $1,221,197

15. Liberty Mutual – $1,120,228

16. American Council of Life Insurers – $1,075,336

17. TigerRisk Partners – $1,061,145

18. Zurich Financial Services – $993,045

19. American Financial Group – $983,176

20. Payroll & Insurance Group – $969,050

Together their contributions amounted to a grand total of $47,986,467.

All donations took place during the 2015–16 election cycle and were released by the Federal Election Commission in May 2017.

OSOCFRP also reported the top twenty recipients:

1. Clinton, Hillary (D) – $2,492,387

2. Trump, Donald (R) – $838,162

3. Rubio, Marco (R-FL), Senate – $669,427

4. Ryan, Paul (R-WI), House – $666,849

5. Cruz, Ted (R-TX), Senate – $661,876

6. Portman, Rob (R-OH), Senate – $626,163

7. Schumer, Charles E (D-NY), Senate – $500,900

8. Toomey, Pat (R-PA), Senate – $499,980

9. Bush, Jeb (R) – $459,822

10. Burr, Richard (R-NC), Senate – $442,675

11. McCarthy, Kevin (R-CA), House – $424,300

12. Scott, Tim (R-SC), Senate – $421,525

13. Tiberi, Patrick J. (R-OH), House – $383,010

14. Wyden, Ron (D-OR), Senate – $377,257

15. Isakson, Johnny (R-GA), Senate – $377,250

16. McHenry, Patrick (R-NC), House – $351,875

17. Neal, Richard E (D-MA), House – $345,700

18. Luetkemeyer, Blaine (R-MO), House – $343,458

19. Crapo, Mike (R-ID), Senate – $326,750

20. Johnson, Ron (R-WI), Senate – $326,273

OSOCFRP reported that annual lobbying on insurance totaled $147,464,746 during the same year. The number of clients reported was 169. The total number of lobbyists reported was 857.

What is a lobbyist? Many people consider a lobbyist an activist who seeks to persuade members of the government (like members of Congress) to enact legislation that will benefit their group.

Although some may not consider lobbyists a legitimate and integral part of our democratic political process, they are needed to change politicians' views on an issue. While most people think of lobbyists only as paid professionals making upward of $300,000 per year, many are volunteers. The average lobbyist may make between $75,000 to $100,000 annually.

In order to be an effective lobbyist, researching and analyzing legislation or regulatory proposals is required. Lobbyists also attend congressional hearings and educate government officials and corporate officers on important issues.

Lobbyists may also use advertising campaigns to change public opinion and the opinion of political leaders.

According to OpenSecrets.org, four out of ten industries that spent the most on lobbyists were in healthcare.

The four areas are pharmaceuticals / health products, $63,168,503; insurance, $38,280,437; hospitals / nursing homes, $23,609,607; and health professionals, $22,175,579.

Pretty shocking numbers, wouldn't you say? That's a lot of money spent on bending the ear and dare I say strong-arming votes from lawmakers. It works like this: Company A gives to candidate B. Candidate B is beholden to company A's interests in future legislation.

Now let's look at how much CEOs of insurance companies and healthcare companies make annually.

In 2016, Fierce Healthcare reported that Michael Neidorff of Centene led the pack of the top eight insurance company salaries. Neidorff earned $22 million in 2016, making him the highest-paid CEO of the largest publicly traded health insurers. His annual earnings were up $1.2 million from 2015.

Humana's Bruce Broussard was the next highest-paid executive at $19.7 million in 2016. What was most surprising about Broussard's salary was his considerable raise of $9.3 million. It marked an increase from 2015 of $10.4 million.

The third-highest-paid CEO was Aetna's Mark Bertolini, earning $18.7 million in 2016, up from $17.3 million. Joseph Swedish, CEO of Anthem, was fourth, earning $16.5 million, up from 2015's $13.6 million.

Although David Cordani, Cigna's CEO, took a pay cut, earning $15.3 million in 2016 compared to $17.3 million in 2015, he was the fifth-highest-paid insurance executive in this study.

J. Mario Molina, the Molina Healthcare CEO, was the sixth-highest-paid insurance company executive, although he, like Cordini, saw his total compensation dip slightly from $10.3 million to $10 million. Cordini and Molina were the only two CEOs to earn less year over year.

UnitedHealth's Stephen Hemsley earned $17.8 million in 2016, an increase from the $14.5 million he earned in 2015, making him the seventh-highest insurance-company-executive earner.

In last place (can we get out the Kleenex, please?), making only $9.3 million in 2016, compared to only $7.8 million the year prior, was Ken Burdick, Wellcare's CEO.

So are you starting to see the money trail? You pay more. You get less. And the companies who take your hard-earned cash get richer.

It gets better.

Let's look at the next list of CEOs from Healthcare Industry companies.

Here are the top twenty earners as compiled by the Associated Press and Equilar, which analyzed CEO pay at hundreds of companies on the S&P 500.

They include the following:

1. Leonard S. Schleifer, Reneger Pharmaceuticals – $47,462,526

2. Jeffrey M. Leiden, Vertex Pharmaceuticals – $28,099,820

3. Larry J. Merlo, CVS Health – $22,855,374

4. Robert J. Hugin, Celgene – $22,472,912

5. Alex Gorsky, Johnson & Johnson – $21,128,866

6. Michael F. Neidorff, Centene – $20,755,103

7. Alan B. Miller, Universal Health Services – $20,427,309

8. Kenneth C. Frazier, Merck & Co. – $19,898,438

9. Miles D. White, Abbott Laboratories – $19,410,704

10. John C. Martin, Gilead Sciences – $18,755,952

11. Richard A. Gonzalez, AbbVie – $18,534,310

12. Heather Bresch, Mylan – $18,162,852

13. David M. Cordani, Cigna – $17,307,672

14. Mark T. Bertolini, Aetna – $17,260,806

15. George A. Scangos, Biogen – $16,874,386

16. Robert L. Parkinson, Baxter International – $16,648,750

17. John C. Lechleiter, Eli Lilly & Co. – $16,562,500

18. Marc N. Casper, Thermo Fisher Scientific – $16,307,079

19. Robert A. Bradway, Amgen – $16,097,714

20. George Paz, Express Scripts Holding – $14,835,587

Total CEO compensation includes salary, bonus, stock and stock option awards, and other perks. It also includes healthcare. Top healthcare—top-of-the-line insurance (ponder that irony) that is unavailable to folks like you and me.

You might as well say some of these CEOs have hit a lotto jackpot without buying a one-dollar ticket. You see, millions of people like you and me are paying thousands in their money game, or jackpot, if you will. And when we need to cash out to protect our own health, our investments are not fully available.

Does the word *greed* start to enter your mind yet?

Who would have thought the biggest money earners in the United States would be healthcare company CEOs? CEOs are just managing a company, right? But for average earnings of $37 million a year.

Let's see how they top out against other industry sectors.

The biggest compensation in ten different industries: Healthcare, followed by information technology, energy, financials, consumer discretionary, industrials, real estate, materials, consumer staples, and finally telecommunications.

Ponder that healthcare comes in ahead of information technology. If that isn't an indication that our priorities are out of whack here, I'm not sure what is.

So, it's the business of medicine that drives medicine, not the steward of it. Comparatively, the best-trained surgeon who has attended at least twelve years of postsecondary education does not make a half a million a year now.

In some instances, healthcare companies are helmed by leaders who began their careers on the front lines of medicine. They include Patricia Hemingway Hall, who is a nurse-turned-executive and who serves as CEO of Blue Cross & Blue Shield of Illinois (she earned $16 million in

2012) and Dr. Belén Garijo, a physician for six years before becoming the president and CEO for Merck Serono, where he earned $6,570,440.

Perhaps there is something to be said for giving up patient care and focusing on managing healthcare cost. Although I'm not sure if the Blue Cross organizations, which began in 1930, ever saw this kind of profit being made in healthcare when they developed the first form of an employer-sponsored hospitalization plan in Texas.

What is more baffling is how it is OK for the politicians to receive money from insurance companies for their campaigns, but not OK for physicians to receive monetary gains for their practices. Both serve our community, right?

Ask yourself this question: do you think insurance companies could be influencing our politicians by donating money to elect them to office?

Before there was an employer-sponsored hospitalization plan, individual hospitals around the nation had begun offering services to individuals on a prepaid basis, eventually leading to the development of Blue Cross organizations. The first employer-sponsored hospitalization plan was created by teachers in Dallas, Texas, in 1929.

Health insurance today is supposed to cover the whole or a part of the risk of a person incurring medical expenses, spreading the risk over a large number of persons. According to the Health Insurance Association of America, health insurance is defined as "coverage that provides for the payments of benefits as a result of sickness or injury. It includes insurance for losses from accident, medical expense, disability, or accidental death and dismemberment."

But the truth of the matter nowadays is that paying for insurance is simply a hedge against good care. The way things are going with an ongoing pattern of denying care, equipment, and tests along with the rising costs, many people are simply giving up. Instead of paying into a pot, they reject insurance altogether, sadly telling themselves that they cannot afford to get sick.

There was a reason why the Obamacare program penalized people on their taxes for not paying into the government system and getting on those exchanges. That system only worked if people were forced into coverage—often coverage that they did not want and in many cases did not need. People wised up—decried having to pay for coverage on things that had nothing to do with them personally—and said no. What is a $90 tax penalty compared to $700 monthly premiums? This has led lawmakers to attempt to fix a significantly flawed system that is more broken than many could have imagined.

Now we see the long, dim view of the plan. Healthcare is now rationed—even for those with insurance coverage. I see it all the time. During my in-service visits with physicians, they tell me that hospital administrators do not want them doing tests anymore after admitting a patient in the hospital. Administrators only want physicians to do surgeries or procedures that bring in the big bucks and then discharge the patients as quickly after their procedures as possible. Several physicians have shared with me that where they practice, it is now frowned upon to run a simple blood test— often a baseline barometer into a health issue. If physicians cannot start there, with a simple blood test, what should you do? Guess.

I am also hearing that some emergency rooms will only treat true emergencies like a heart attack. If you go to the ER for something less than a big issue, the staff will check your vital signs, order a blood test, a urinalysis, and maybe even an

X-ray to determine your servility. If you are stable, the ER will discharge you and advise you to see a primary care physician. If you need a specialist, like a cardiologist, your primary physician can refer you.

In this conundrum, it is no wonder many people simply get their healthcare needs at a doc-in-the-box walk-in clinic. It is fast, it is often cheaper, and they can get something painful or annoying like a UTI or a respiratory infection treated quickly—before it becomes a bigger deal.

Healthcare likes to sidestep the process. If indeed you are able to see the primary care physician for your issue, after being examined by your physician, and if he or she determines from running a series of tests that you need be admitted to the hospital for a procedure or surgery, then he or she will begin the paperwork needed.

By keeping these steps outside the hospital setting in the beginning, the rationale is that it will save hospitals and insurance companies a huge amount of money. The average cost of a day in the hospital is now between $4,000 to $5,000.

The ER, where many of us turned for immediate care, is no longer admitting patients to the hospital unless you truly need to be admitted. ERs are no longer doing extensive testing either. This is a new healthcare custom causing outrage in communities. Most people have been trained to go to the ER, and if you call your physician's office after hours, chances are you will hear a recording advising you to go to the ER if you have an emergency.

Who gets penalized in this equation? Typically our most vulnerable. Older folks who do not have a car or insurance will go to the ER when they are at the point of no return.

If you are thinking the skilled nursing facility can drive an older patient to the ER, that is true, but according to an article on WebMD, only 11 percent of patients over sixty-five years old live in a skilled nursing facility.

Will we begin to see the ER deny nonacute patients care because they do not have a primary physician or health insurance? Who is liable if a patient gets discharged and dies after leaving?

This protocol must be fixed. Money must not be allowed to take precedence over health. Even in our political divide, I think we can all agree to that.

We have in place in our country a process that offers prisoners who are incarcerated better access to treatment than many Americans who are law-abiding. We lock them up in the name of justice and provide them with food, shelter, clothes, an education, a place to work out, and healthcare. It is basic human rights, activists admonish.

And yet...not for the rest of us.

As it stands now in the United States, inmates have more opportunities than many of us who have not broken the law.

Let's look at the math. According to the Prison Policy Initiative website, there are more than two million people in US prisons. Our American criminal justice system is holding more than 2.3 million inmates in 1,719 state prisons, 102 federal prisons, 942 juvenile correction facilities, 3,283 local jails, and 79 Indian-country jails and in military prisons. We are not even counting the immigration-detention facilities, civil commitment centers, and other US territories.

And you, in addition to the high premiums and high deductibles you are paying, also through your taxes, give care to people who frankly deserve it far less than you do.

For all of these reasons, I do not know why our politicians are so allergic to a single-payer healthcare system unless they are not patriotic. I am also not sure why we do not have faith in a single-payer system. We already have two forms of socialized medicine, called Medicare and Medicaid. And you know what would happen if we discontinued either or both of those. People would be up in arms!

According to the Henry J. Kaiser Family Foundation, 17.6 million (33 percent) of beneficiaries were enrolled in a Medicare Advantage plan in 2016. Medicare Advantage plans pay for out-of-pocket charges. About 69 percent—55,504,005 million people—were enrolled in traditional Medicare in 2017.

Medicaid had 68,884,085 million enrolled, while our Children's Health Insurance Program had 5,646,917 million enrolled in April 2017. That figure was up 29 percent from 2016. Most people do not know or understand the Center for Medicare and Medicaid Services (CMS) sets the rates for medical products and services reimbursement. Private commercial insurance follows the reimbursement rates CMS sets.

Another important fact most Americans do not know or understand is an individual can be dually enrolled in Medicare and Medicaid. It is our American taxes that support these programs—both state and federal taxes.

So why not a single-payer system? Most of us are already paying taxes for millions of people to have healthcare. Why not us, too? We need to put our outrage over our healthcare system to work and create a program that would eliminate corporate greed and corruption in our politics.

Over sixteen countries have a single-payer system, including Norway, Japan, the United Kingdom, Kuwait, Sweden, Bahrain, Brunei, Canada, the United Arab Emirates, Finland, Slovenia, Italy, Portugal, Cyprus, Spain, and Iceland.

Some of my friends from Germany and Switzerland, who live in New York City now, claim when it comes to nonemergency and elective surgery, Germany and Switzerland have faster access than the United States. As with our educational system, it seems our health programs are now slipping when compared to our friends around the world. We can and should do better.

So is greed from our politicians and corporate America keeping you and me from a single-payer system? Don't get me wrong. I am not looking for anyone to take care of me. I like my healthcare system that I have created for myself. I take personal responsibility for my role in keeping me healthy.

However, should I or any other American need acute healthcare, I know our country could create a single-payer healthcare system for a lot less with a better, more humane quality of care.

A single-payer system is not the same thing as socialized medicine, as many like to assert. I am not suggesting our government should control hospitals or healthcare employees or healthcare providers, nor am I suggesting eliminating lawsuits. I am suggesting a single-payer system where every person in this country could get healthcare without losing his or her job or home.

The two-cent national healthcare sales tax would work regardless if you were covered or not. We are already paying for uninsured patients with our high premiums and with the help of state and federal taxes. Why not be transparent about the total cost of care and the greed behind healthcare in our country?

Last year, *Forbes* magazine's website reported that Americans would spend over $1 trillion on Christmas gifts between November 2016 and January 2017. Within three months of Christmas shopping, we spent at least 25 percent of healthcare costs in the United States—on our Christmas gifts. This proves this healthcare tax program could work.

While some will say, "I don't want to pay for other people to get the same healthcare." I have news for them. You already are. Who do you think pays for patients who are admitted to the hospital without insurance? Our tax dollars.

And finally, let me raise this point: our world outside of the hospital has helped to make relationships transactional, rather than relational.

A transactional relationship means exactly what it sounds like. I only call on my neighbor when I need something or a favor. For instance, I hear he is going to the World Series, and I ask him to bring me back a souvenir.

Relational means creating a mutual caring friendship. I notice my neighbor's car is in the garage later than normal. I call over to see how my neighbor is doing, and he says he feels too sick to get up out of bed. I then ask him if he needs anything from the store, like Gatorade, offering my neighbor friendship. I then ask if he needs help walking his dog.

These are old customs most of our neighbors enjoyed in the sixties and seventies, when I was growing up. My parents instilled these values in me. And it was simple: to care for others, to help others when they needed help.

People today are too busy being selfish, no longer spending quality time with one another to get to know one another as human beings—placing material needs and money before friendship.

Is there any reason to think our healthcare system is going to be different if we are not?

Without our health, we have nothing. Why not create a system that is proactive, not reactive, and rewards Americans for making healthier choices and thoughtful decisions about the care they want to pay for and need?

We can do better. I truly believe there is a way ahead.

Chapter 10

Losing It All

Shortly after moving to New York in 1998, I remember visiting my brother-in-law's mother, Zelda. Zelda was a widow. Her husband, Marty, was an ob-gyn for many years before he died.

I used to smile during my visits with Zelda when she would answer her phone, "Dr. Malachowsky's residence." Then I would hear that on the line was so-and-so, "a Marty baby."

We would then go to lunch at the local deli in Oakhurst, New Jersey, and everyone would gladly greet Zelda. "Hello, Mrs. Malachowsky," they would say. And Zelda would then tell me "that person was a Marty baby;" afterward, she would point out about six more eating in the deli.

Zelda was proud to be a doctor's wife. She raised their sons while he worked, sharing him with other women who needed his skills so they, too, could be moms with healthy babies.

I learned many wonderful things from Zelda. Three of the most interesting things I learned were her thoughts on the wrong direction our healthcare was headed, what patients could tell us, and the importance of relationships.

Zelda graduated from Columbia College with a master's degree in occupational therapy (OT). She gave up her career as an OT in 1955 to marry Martin Malachowsky and to become a mother.

"I was taught if you listen to the patient long enough…they will tell you what's going on in their bodies," Zelda would often say, every time we spoke about an obstetric patient who was on my high-risk obstetrics company's service.

If a patient didn't have insurance or enough money to cover their bills, Marty would allow them to "square up" by making payments or trading goods or services equal to the bill, she said.

"Now insurance companies have total control as to how much the provider receives and the patient has to pay, regardless if it creates hardships for both," Zelda said.

Zelda and Marty had two couples they vacationed with during the year. All of the men (husbands) were physicians, and the women (doctors' wives) were stay-at-home moms.

Each husband was a physician in a different modality. Marty, of course, was the ob-gyn; Al, an internal medicine physician; and Sam, a surgeon.

Shaking her head, Zelda said, "I can remember when Marty got a phone call in the early seventies from a lobbyist wanting to represent him and other ob-gyns against managed care."

According to Zelda, her husband, Marty, and his colleagues were so busy taking care of their patients that they overlooked the importance of the issue—a mistake that would end up haunting Marty and other physicians a few years later.

In 1973, Congress passed the Health Maintenance Organization Act, which encouraged the rapid growth of health maintenance organizations, the first form of managed care.

And now, forty-four years later, we have this huge crisis in our healthcare system that no one can fix, not even our politicians.

You see, even though we have made huge strides in medical advancements to improve remission rates to prolong lives with many cancers today, we have not closed the gaps in the cost associated with patients and their families, who are often left to pay an enormous 20 percent co-payment.

My late friend Michael Conmy knew this game firsthand, how 20 percent can add up fast and become a hefty sum for patients like him. Mike had been fighting pulmonary sarcoma for several years, and although he thought his insurance was pretty good, his co-pay soared to over a quarter of a million dollars before he died in August 2017. Medical bills from serious illnesses can add up to the cost of most Americans homes—a giant sum, but one that Mike's estate is now responsible for after his heroic battle against cancer.

Ponder Mike's story, and ask yourself if our current healthcare system really works. Honestly. Losing your job. Your home for your family to live in. Your life?

Who do you think pays for Mike and other folks in his shoes if they cannot pay the balance? Precisely—you and me. Our tax dollars at work. Taxes created from the politicians we elected. Politicians who have the 2017 Bentley of insurance plans compared to the 1969 Volkswagen Beetle that you and I have.

Mike, my friend and former colleague, who died at forty-seven, was a type 1 diabetic. He was diagnosed in November 2015 with pulmonary sarcoma. Mike was also a registered nurse, a former co-founder of a subcutaneous-insulin-pump company, a devoted husband of sixteen years, a father of four (ages three to thirteen years old), a brother, and a son. Never in his wildest dreams did he think what his turn being cared for as a patient with a life-threatening disease would be and that it would be this early in his life. Neither did his wife, Marie, who is an occupational therapist like Zelda.

Mike's cancer symptoms began with a simple cough and a rash he found on his foot before we left for new-hire training with our negative-pressure wound-therapy company.

He had heard I had missed a day of work after having vaccines required by my work. I felt nauseated and noticed a rash on the side of my stomach, which was a common side effect from the vaccines I had been given.

Mike was hoping that his own rash was a similar side effect from the same vaccines.

Unfortunately, after further testing by his physician, this was not the case.

Mike called me that afternoon to tell me the news of what his physician discovered was the primary cause of his rash: pulmonary sarcoma, stage IIIB.

His odds were not the best, but his cancer did not realize the person it had invaded. Mike Conmy was a fighter and a man of faith, with a fearless champion and wife by his side. Marie, along with thousands from his community, began to join his journey, and we stood by him until the end.

Everyone who heard the news of his early diagnosis knew how devastating this was and how scary for him and his family because he was the primary breadwinner.

We each pitched in, taking turns stopping by to check on Mike, Marie, and the kids. These cheerleaders would cook meals, clean, shuttle kids, raise money, whatever was needed to keep Mike moving toward remission.

In January 2017, Mike's cancer returned, literally inside his heart, which is very rare. He knew this development would force him to give up his job and further imperil his family financially.

After this news, I stopped by for a cup of tea with Mike. He always enjoyed boiling water and making me a cup of Irish tea.

We would sit, and I would listen to him tell me beautiful stories of each of his kids and how wonderful Marie was in keeping him going.

He shared how tough it was to get out of bed some days because the pain was so great; it was difficult to stand. The vomiting he was experiencing from his chemotherapy also hindered him tremendously in being able to talk to insurance companies, who denied coverage for medications he needed.

Many times, with tears in his eyes, I would listen to him say he did not understand how folks our parents' age could handle health insurance companies in modern times with computers, websites, and cell phone applications. I knew my dad could not.

Mike had to reach out to his local congressman to get help with his insurance-company coverage. Almost immediately after his congressman, US Representative Sean Patrick Maloney, and his US senator William J. Larkins called on Mike's behalf, the Conmy landline would ring with approval from the insurance company. It was as if these lawmakers had magical powers after Mike had spent days on the phone being constantly denied while he fought for his life.

One day, after our visit, I left Mike's house and headed to a hospital in Westchester County, New York. My colleague and I had an appointment with the program director at the wound-care center to review ordering some of our advanced wound dressings.

The program director shared with us that one of her patients who was treated with our epidermal-harvesting system had been discharged before we walked in. This patient had a stubborn, chronic four-year-old wound that would not heal. For three years prior to my colleague and I in-servicing the wound-care-center physicians on our epidermal-harvesting system, this patient could not even get a shoe over his right foot, which also meant he could not walk. He had to use a wheelchair.

As we all showed our enthusiasm for this patient, we also knew that older patients who live in an assisted living facility, and who cannot drive, get desperately needed social contact when they come to facilities to be treated. The program director then expressed concern for her patient.

Apparently, this happens more often than not because most children of older folks park their parents in a skilled-nursing facility, rarely returning to visit. We all get caught up in life's pressures and trying to make ends meet. Although it may not be our intention, "out of sight, out of mind" happens. Time flies for us, but not for our parents, who are alone.

After sharing this sad conundrum, we began to focus on the business at hand. I asked her about co-pays. Somehow, we managed to get on the topic of my former colleague and how his own co-pays were wreaking havoc in his life.

The program director explained that healthcare providers had nothing to do with the rates negotiated for patients by the insurance companies, yet the patients are held responsible and are not allowed to "square up" the way Zelda described earlier.

This is what leaves patients with enormous amounts of healthcare cost not covered by their insurance companies, which puts tons of pressure on older individuals who can no longer work, she told me.

"Some patients don't even know what they signed up for, and others try to avoid what they're signed up for with payers like Medicare," said the program director.

She shared a story about one of her patients from a few years ago. Apparently, this seventy-year-old male patient was from back in the old days, where people had pride and would not accept "handouts" or "charity care." This patient insisted on meeting his financial obligation solely on his own merits.

This patient was so emphatic about staying ahead of his medical bills he followed them all. The program director said he would call wanting to know why something was still owed. If something was still owed, legitimately or not, he wanted to know why he had something outstanding.

He was a guy who took pride in always paying his own way. One day the program director and his doctor noticed he started not wanting to come to his appointments. She figured she needed to talk to him to see what was going on.

The program director convinced her patient and his wife to come in for a meaningful talk about his bills. After the couple agreed to come to the office and talk with her, they got a bill from the hospital, and they did not understand why.

The patient had been going to the wound-care center, and all his bills had been paid by Medicare. He thought there was no out-of-pocket to him. Everything was supposed to be covered.

However, after his last visit, something changed. The program director told him that she was not aware they had done anything differently. The patient explained that the last couple of times he came for a doctor's appointment, he got a bill. The healthcare bill stated that he still owed money, and he told the program director he did not have that kind of money because he lives on a fixed income.

The patient went on to say he did not want to come to the wound-care center and not meet his financial obligations, which the program director told him she could totally understand and appreciate.

The program director said she looked him in the eye and said, "We're billing you the same thing we billed you when you came all the other times, and now it's not covered? I really don't understand that—there has to be a mistake. Something is wrong."

She added, "I don't know where the charge is coming from, but from everything I can see, this is not going to cost you anything."

But this patient was so entrenched in meeting his financial obligation that he stopped coming to his appointments. Then his doctors said to the program director, you have got to get him back here.

So, upon the request from his doctor, she started calling this patient. When she finally reached him, she pleaded for him to return, assuring him that the payment would be OK. He finally agreed, and then the patient's doctor wanted to do a procedure on him that would require the man to incur a hospital stay.

The patient informed her, "Absolutely not, absolutely not." He told her he did not want to owe any more money.

However, as time passed and after several conversations between him and his wife, the man agreed. He was admitted to the hospital, and the procedure was completed. Then, the patient's doctor had to go out of town that weekend for a medical conference.

When the patient found out his doctor would be out of town over the weekend, he asked if he could be discharged before his doctor left. The patient's reasoning was that he did not want to have to be in the hospital all weekend and incur any more costs than were necessary. So, the doctor agreed to discharge him before leaving town.

During the time between his hospital discharge and his

next office appointment, which was the following Tuesday, the physician reached out to the wound-care program director, asking her to call and check in on his patient. When she called, she found out the patient had killed himself at home.

The patient's wife told the program director that her husband was so distraught over what he might owe, he could not take it anymore. He did not want to leave her or his kids with an unbearable amount of healthcare bills to pay off.

With tears in her eyes as she finished telling this patient's tragic story, the program director quickly picked herself up and explained that this man was unique. Many other patients who visit the clinic could care less how much it would cost.

According to the program director, some patients don't want to pay or can't pay because it would mean going without other necessities, such as food or shelter. She explained that some patients in that situation expect to still receive healthcare, regardless of their financial responsibility.

She then continued to explain that is why losses and profits are so critical for hospitals and facilities.

"We don't have any state or federal money bailing us out," she said. "I'm responsible for the bottom line."

My conversation with her identified one of the biggest problems in our healthcare system—so many people are coming from different places, with different understandings of how our healthcare system actually works.

"I try to inform the patient so the patient can make an informed choice," she said. "This is the only way I can see this place existing, and the only way to do that is to inform them about their 20 percent co-pay responsibility."

According to the program director, some people do not want to pay. They just expect you to give it to them, regardless of their financial responsibility.

Well, that may be true for some but not one of our company's NPWT patients whom I met last summer.

Shieva was the same age as Mike, forty-seven. She too has a spouse and three kids ages five to thirteen years old. She is also a healthcare professional. In fact, she is a physician, an ob-gyn with a large practice. She was voted "Ob-gyn of the Year" where she practices. She is the breadwinner in her family and is working while receiving treatment for stage II ovarian cancer.

Although she is trying to convince me she is working part-time by her standards, she is really full time by corporate America's. And not once does she complain or say anything derogatory or negative. Victim is not a role in her story. Every moment spent by her is meaningful and relished.

Weeks after she was discharged from our services, her insurance denied partial payment for her NPWT. Really? While she's fighting for her life, they want her to argue about whose responsibility it is to cover her NPWT outside of the hospital, saving her payers thousands of dollars in hospitalization costs should she have been admitted?

And yes, she would have been admitted because she had an infection in her wound.

This is one of many games in our healthcare system that has to stop. The only way it will stop is with a single-payer system, where we all get the same quality of care at the same cost, no matter who we are or what we do.

We have to demand a single-payer system. Healthcare is our right, and if we unite around this cause, we have power.

Chapter 11

Replacing Obamacare

On a hot Thursday morning, July 20th, 2017, as soon as I finished my daily meditation, prayers, and ACIM ("A Course in Miracles") lesson, I received a voicemail to call my colleague Kristi Means.

Before returning her call, I reflected on the day's lesson, number 206: "I am not a body. I am free. For I am still as God created me."

I had been hearing this quote for a few days and was questioning the repetition.

Kristi is my soul sister and a miracle baby. I dubbed her "soul sister" because we have similar values when it comes to life and political views concerning America—"miracle baby" because she truly is a miracle.

To look at our outer appearances, I am considered white and Kristi black. However, our skin does not stop our hearts from connecting or working together.

Kristi would tease me about how hard it is to call her black because I was brought up not to refer to people by the color of their skin but by their name.

Kristi and I created the nonprofit Sisters for Liberty. As women, we know what it feels like to grow up as a minority, which fueled our fire to do more than the average person by teaching civics and American history and to stand up for healthcare for all under a single-payer system.

I call her a "miracle baby" because years ago, before her mother, Mrs. Robinson, knew she was pregnant with Kristi, Mrs. Robinson had thought she had her tubes tied, preventing her from being pregnant.

However, Mrs. Robinson was feeling a lot of the familiar symptoms she had felt six times before while being pregnant with Kristi's siblings.

Mrs. Robinson called her ob-gyn, the physician who had delivered all of her babies and who had also "tied her tubes"— so they thought. Mrs. Robinson's physician told her there was no way she could be pregnant because he remembered her surgery years before.

Before hanging up the phone, the physician humored Mrs. Robinson by scheduling an appointment to run a blood test. Sure enough, after the test results came back positive, Mrs. Robinson was right. She knew her body well; she was pregnant.

On January 1 of the following year, Mrs. Robinson gave birth to Kristi Michelle, her miracle baby. A miracle because when a woman has her tubes tied, it is to prevent a pregnancy.

As I play back Kristi's voicemail message, I can hear the excitement in her voice saying, "I think I have a patient you're going to want to meet."

His name was George Scombulis. She told me that she had already talked to him about me and my book project. It was significant, she said, because in her view he was truly one of the only people she had met who had benefited from the Affordable Care Act. Leave it to my "miracle baby" to find a "miracle man."

His doctors called him a "walking miracle" because, by medical standards, he would have been dead three years ago had it not been for his insurance program.

"I wouldn't be alive today if it weren't for Obamacare," he said.

Before Scombulis was diagnosed with systemic scleroderma, his physician thought that severe allergies were causing his skin problems. He asked Scombulis to get rid of his dog, furniture, and clothes, to sand his wooden floors and revarnish them, and to stop drinking beer and consuming sugar.

Well, getting rid of his dog, a giant schnauzer named Malcolm, was not an option because he loved him so much and could not bear letting him go—until the day Scombulis's house caught on fire, and he lost everything the physician had suggested.

Heartbroken and homeless, Scombulis was miffed. He knew a higher power had to have had a hand in this in order for him to live, although Scombulis did not call this power God. The fire inspector told Scombulis the fire was started by reversed polarity due to very old wiring in the house. The house had been built in 1870, and the wiring had never been updated.

Scombulis had endured so much. In the beginning, Scombulis's face was enlarged ten times its normal size, making him unrecognizable to his friends and loved ones. "My face was morphed, and my skin was discolored with patterns resembling camouflage," said Scombulis. "I was a human photobomb and felt like I looked like a monster with gorilla hands."

Imagine only wanting to wear pants or shirts that pull on or over because buttons are too painful or complicated for your sore, blistered fingers. Scombulis now wears shoes that slide on or that have straps, not laces, because his disease has compromised his dexterity. If he gets invited out to dinner, he has a pair of dress slacks with his belt already threaded through the pants' belt loops so he can easily slide into them without too much trouble. He has mastered using his dining utensils after lots of practice in fear he would fling food everywhere and not be asked out again.

Over the last twenty-four years, Scombulis has lost almost everything but his life, exploring his options and treatment plan around the country. He traveled to Harvard, Johns Hopkins, San Francisco, Hartford, NYU, and Yale. Fortunately, he had friends or relatives who lived in these towns, making it feasible for him to gather as much knowledge as he could about what was going on with his body.

The only thing Scombulis knew for sure was that whatever he had was rare and life-threatening.

Finally, Scombulis was diagnosed on October 6, 1993, with systemic scleroderma. Systemic scleroderma is a group of autoimmune diseases that change the skin, blood vessels, muscles and internal organs. He looks similar to a burn victim in places on his body.

Kristi described Scombulis as a modern-day Henrietta Lacks, with the exception that Scombulis had given written consent to use his cells for research. Lacks, whose life was chronicled in a book and soon-to-be movie helmed by Oprah Winfrey, had no prior knowledge, nor did she give consent to use her cells in research.

Scombulis is aware of Lacks's story and the positive and profound impact her cells had in helping the medical community and patients. He hopes to help others with his cells by sharing his experience of living with this horrific disease.

In deep admiration and appreciation of her cells, Scombulis goes on to share what he knew about Lacks's contributions to the medical world.

Lacks was an African American woman whose cancer cells

were the source of the HeLa cell line, the first immortalized cell line and one of the most important cell lines in medical research. Her cells were named after the *He* in *Henrietta* and the *La* in *Lacks*.

The HeLa cell is an immortalized cell line that will reproduce indefinitely under specific conditions, and the HeLa cell line continues to be a source of invaluable medical data to the present day. Many modern-day products use her cells in skin substitutes, in vitro. The Lacks family was not aware of the HeLa cell line until 1975 and was never compensated for the extractions of her cells.

George Otto Gey was the first researcher to study Lacks's cancerous cells. Gey observed that her cells were unique in that they reproduced at a very high rate and could be kept alive long enough to allow more in-depth examination.

For this reason, Lacks's is the oldest and most commonly used human cell line. These were the first human cells grown in a lab that were naturally "immortal," meaning that they would not die after a set number of cell divisions (i.e., lack of senescence).

The HeLa cell was used by virologists to study viruses. Its uses are widespread.

Lacks's cells helped researchers not only understand methods of freezing cells for storage and of standardizing methods for culturing cells, but were also used to develop the first polio vaccine, and were a template for accurately determining the number of chromosomes in cells.

The cells were also hugely beneficial for cancer research and were used to study effects of radiation as well as the effects of deep-sea pressure and the safety of cosmetics and pharmaceuticals.

In addition, Lacks's cells allowed scientists to replace lab animals, used for research on HIV, the most common sexually transmitted disease, and to help with developing treatments for AIDS.

The cells have also been used in researching what causes aging, in studying the effects of salmonella and tuberculosis, in determining that HPV causes cancer, and to help develop treatments for Parkinson's disease, influenza, leukemia, and hemophilia.

Broadly, Lacks's contributions to medicine are staggering.

Lacks's body was buried near her mother's, without a tombstone, in October 1951. Roland Pattillo, a faculty member of the Morehouse School of Medicine, and who had worked with Gey Pattillo, knew the Lacks family and felt for them and their loss.

Pattillo donated a headstone in the shape of a book, and it contains an epitaph written by her grandchildren.

It reads:

Henrietta Lacks

August 1, 1920–October 4, 1951
　　In loving memory of a phenomenal woman, wife and mother who touched the lives of many. Here lies Henrietta Lacks (HeLa). Her immortal cells will continue to help mankind forever.
　　Eternal Love and Admiration, From Your Family.

Back to Scombulis, whose cells are also helping researchers.

Yale scientists are making improved mouse models with his cells. Yale had used traditional mouse models that ran on mouse DNA. After eleven years of work, Yale scientists developed a line of mice whose immune systems were totally wiped out. After altering the mouse's immune system, scientists could inject human DNA.

Instead of using a petri dish, which would mimic our human body's systems, Yale created a human-system environment inside a mouse's body by eradicating or overtaking the mouse's natural immune system—with Scombulis's cells.

Now, Scombulis says, "My physicians at Yale are injecting my cells into some of these mice. So when you do a test on the mice, you will get the human response, not the mouse's response. This is better than a mouse's response for a human because although the human brain and immune system are similar to the mouse's, test results can be different."

Yale calls it "humanizing" mice by injecting them with human cells from Scombulis. It will allow them to do further research developing cures for diseases like his.

Currently, Yale pays Scombulis $100 for each skin sample and $500 per bone marrow extraction. According to Scombulis, he and his physicians will know more on the success when they see the results of his latest tests.

"My cells are the first test model," he said. "I'm living my moral obligation to our society by donating my cells."

Scumbulis and his doctors are not sure what caused his systemic scleroderma.

It took thirty-seven physicians to diagnose him twenty-four years ago. They believe that his disease could have been caused by genetics or environmental factors.

The physicians who care for Scombulis have not been able to prove yet that it is caused by genetics. No one in his family has ever been diagnosed with systemic scleroderma.

However, Scombulis does believe it can be caused by environmental risks because four adults he knows that he grew up with on the same peninsula in Norwalk, Connecticut, have been diagnosed with scleroderma.

As someone living with a chronic condition, he fears what

will happen now that President Trump has rejected a ban on potentially harmful insecticides in our environment, along with other environmental regulations that are in limbo.

Scombulis, who has learned much about his body and medicine, understands that our largest human organ is our skin.

Yale wanted to use a process called photopheresis on Scombulis. Photopheresis is a process where his blood would be withdrawn from the body and zapped with a light. The blood would be treated with a photosensitizing agent and subsequently irradiated with specified wavelengths of light and then reinjected into his body to achieve a positive effect on his skin.

After agreeing to this procedure, Scombulis discovered the cost for his procedure would be $150,000. He did not have insurance or a job with an income. He could barely afford food every day. In fact, he volunteered at the food pantry in Norwalk, Connecticut so he would be assured a good, hearty meal.

He had already spent his life's savings and burned through $70,000 of his retirement mutual funds on blood tests and other medical expenses.

It did not take him long to realize the only answer for him to be able to afford the treatment he needed was to sell his house.

So he sold it to his accountant, who was aware of his circumstances. The accountant agreed to allow Scombulis to stay in his house despite their transaction. When he finally had the money and called to schedule his first treatment, the cost for his procedure had risen to $250,000—more than doubling during the length of time it took him to sell— because of the advances scientists had made in improving photopheresis treatments in the interim.

When Scombulis hung up the phone, in shock at how much his treatment was now going to cost, he started to feel hopeless.

As fate would have it, he noticed that he had a wound on his leg. He went to the Norwalk Wound Care Center to have it examined. It was there that he finally qualified for Medicaid and coverage under the Affordable Care Act. He had tried several times to get on the government program and was turned down because he had earned too much money in the past.

"I think our government thought I was hiding money because I was articulate and white," he said. "My clothes are ragged, my shoes are worn, and I'm in so much pain; it's all I can do to stand."

He added, "There must be a God because of all of the synchronicity I'm experiencing. What are the chances I'd get Obamacare when I literally had no other option? I have no living family. My mom is gone, and so is my sister."

Now he is able to continue his photopheresis treatments. Are they working? Scombulis says he cannot see a "damn thing" on the outside, but he is told by his physicians that the treatments are working on the inside.

"I must be getting better because when I ride on the train, people actually will allow me to sit by them," Scombulis said. "Before I was diagnosed, if I'd ride the train to New York City, people would get up as soon as I sat next to them. They'd rather stand than to sit next to me looking like a monster."

Scombulis says that if Congress and President Trump repeal Obamacare, he will probably commit suicide. Without treatment, Scombulis becomes septic, with infections in his blood.

Although he seems to be getting better with time, he continues to live a life of a lone ranger—and one who misses companionship and who is not able to do much.

"Think about all you do with your hands that I can't do

because of my disease," said Scombulis. "Sports like softball, walk a dog on a leash, play guitar, be a lover. I miss having a girlfriend."

Scombulis continues to battle his disease while living alone in Connecticut, with his closest friends in Europe. The telephone, computer, and visits once in a blue moon act like a lifeline for him to his friends. He claims to take one day at a time. And to insist to persist, never taking his body for granted just because it may look weird. He takes pride in trying to preserve the body he has without knowing what the next step will be.

Scombulis's struggle makes me ponder my own health journey. I now understand the lesson I heard during my ACIM download. Had I not heard that lesson before meeting Scombulis, I might have focused on his body instead of his spirit. Had I done that, I would have missed a great gift. Scombulis is courageous and doesn't allow himself to become his disease.

Chapter 12

Keeping Your Mind Healthy

Reflecting on my life up to this point, I hear two common phrases from my mom that still stick with me.

One is "life is so short," and the other is "your body is your temple."

As a young child, I'd watch my mom preparing healthful gourmet meals for our family. She would swim laps and take long walks in the morning after she would see my father off to work with a hug, kiss, and a bagged lunch she'd prepared for him while he dressed.

My mom looked amazing in a pair of jeans. Being able to look great in a pair of blue jeans was a sign for southern men that you were a "hottie." Looking back, I can see now why she turned heads.

Her daily ritual was putting on a pair of blue jeans, some red lipstick, and a pair of diamond earrings. No other makeup was required, and rarely would you see her wearing any nail polish. She was a natural beauty and believed in always presenting herself as well-dressed and well-groomed in public.

Mom also taught my siblings and me about manners and proper etiquette. She would often refer to Emily Post, who wrote *Etiquette in Society*, and to Judith Martin, known by her pen name, "Miss Manners."

Mom agreed with Post that manners are a sensitive awareness of others.

At the end of Mom's day, she would teach us kids how to give her back rubs, which later became full-body massages—then, how to draw a hot tub bath with bubbles celebrating our day and decorating our souls. This was her way of honoring her body as her temple.

When I first heard her say I needed to start treating my body as a temple so it would last longer and serve me better, I was a teenager.

As a teen, I remember a week seemed like an eternity. And nothing or even the amount of what I put into my body seemed to matter, particularly as far as gaining weight or causing diabetes. Even as I did not care, I had no physical signs showing up in my body that I was eating poorly or treating it badly.

Now I know differently. When it comes to our body, we each have to take responsibility for keeping it fine-tuned. A friend, Maxine Carr, who has a Ph.D. in family therapy, shared with me that "responsibility" simply means the ability to respond with love.

Putting things in our body that would be healthful and loving is how I interpreted it. Comfort foods, I now know, can also be healthful and loving at the same time.

I also realize now that our bodies are our temple. Think of our bodies as the vehicle that transports our mind, thoughts, and spirits.

It is so important to choose healthy thoughts—being careful what we allow into our minds—because our bodies can wreak havoc. Louise Hay and Caroline Myss talk about this in several of their books. Many other authors have written about this as well.

Physicians are starting to recognize the connection too. And as such, more consumers are starting to get this message.

I was pretty lucky. My parents knew from the start: I was "that" kid they had to keep busy through art and sports. I loved both and was fortunate to grow up when I did during the sixties and seventies. I'm still growing.

Back then, in a different era, our school systems seemed to support the body, mind, and spirit connection better with school-funded programs. They abundantly supported the arts, whether music or visual arts like painting or sculpturing. Schools provided a balanced meal at lunch for thirty-five cents a day (and no, you could not buy sodas at school in most places). Our lunches always had plenty of vegetables, meat as the main protein source, a dessert, and a carton of milk.

I can remember loving middle school when I attended Howard Bishop in Gainesville, Florida. It was terrific because we had so many life-experience classes exposing us to our future adulthood, giving a sneak preview of how to care for ourselves after leaving our parents' nest.

We also had classes in home economics, where we learned the importance of a balanced meal and how to create one. Trust me, Mom had already exposed my brother, sisters, and me to this reality. She believed in teamwork and equal opportunity for all in our house. I knew I would ace this course thanks to Mom and her work ethic.

Last May, my brother-in-law, Dale, and my sister Tammy came to visit me. We were all curious about the Culinary Institute of America in Hyde Park, New York. The CIA is only fifteen miles from my house. After deciding on which restaurant we wanted to go to, I made reservations. We chose the student-run Italian, a restaurant called Ristorante Caterina de' Medici.

Keep in mind, some of these students will become a future "chef of America." After all, Anthony Bourdain was a graduate. So how can anyone go wrong with enjoying a wonderful culinary adventure here?

Well, little did we know that it was the first night of the semester that the Ristorante Caterina de' Medici had been open.

We ordered an appetizer, which came promptly. Then the eternal wait began. We noticed other diners were getting anxious for their main entrées as well.

Tammy and Dale had been to several culinary programs throughout the world and had never had to wait this long. The three of us, out of boredom and starvation, saw the comment/feedback card on our table and began to fill it out.

After rereading our feedback, we decided it might be gentler to go and speak to the supervising instructor.

This is when we discovered this was the first time ever some of the students had cooked. Tammy and I were in shock, both reflecting on when we started cooking in our home as children. Mind-blowing to fathom anyone who was eighteen or older had never cooked a meal. Perhaps our educational system in America is depriving our youngsters of important life skills. I mean, what good is an education if you cannot take care of yourself?

In home economics, we had to go shopping and do a cost comparison to find out which grocery store offered the best prices for our wallets. We were learning how to stretch a dollar. After school, our parents would take us to Publix, Winn-Dixie, and A&P, all local food stores within five miles of our house.

In addition to learning how to cook a balanced meal, home economics also reinforced Mom's teachings on how important it was to protect our bodies with clothes. We each learned how to sew an outfit. Most students chose to make a shirt. Frankly, it seemed easy enough, even then.

In middle school, I also enjoyed going to agricultural engineering, where my classmates and I grew a vegetable garden together. I still to this day practice that on my land. My neighbors and I share our harvest and plan our vegetable crops based on what the other is growing. It connects us and nourishes us all in the best way.

Industrial arts was also a required class. Here I learned how to make a cutting board, which is still being used by my father forty years later to cut meat before cooking.

Although my classmates and I were still a few years from driving a car by ourselves, mechanical engineering taught us how to change the oil in our car engines and to change tires.

All of these courses were great to learn in middle school; however, my favorites were physical education and music.

PE was required every year in school until I started high school. Then we were only required for two years. If I took it in my freshman and sophomore years, I was technically done. However, I chose to continue taking PE as a source of movement, not only for my body but also for my soul (mind and thoughts). It was my main outlet where I kept my body looking lean and my spirit feeling energized.

If I ever woke up for school feeling sore from physical exercise, I'd hear my sister Melody's voice saying, "Motion is the lotion. Keep it moving."

I can remember watching a movie on television about Knute Rockne, the Notre Dame Fighting Irish football college head coach from 1918 to 1930. He was the first coach I saw teaching the body-mind-spirit connection—although in sports, he is better known for pioneering the forward pass.

Rockne instilled in his players the value of taking care of

ourselves off the field. He demanded good grades, community service, and civil conduct. Rockne himself was a chemist and a pharmacist, graduating in 1914 from Notre Dame. During his thirteen years of coaching, he led his team to 105 victories, only twelve losses, five ties, and three national championships, including five undefeated seasons without a tie.

So, it looks to me that this old pharmacist took some hints he learned in medicine in the early 1900s and applied them to football. Judging by his football team's record, it worked in sports, too!

The next day at practice, I shared this movie with my coach, and she smiled.

In high school, I continued playing on our softball and basketball teams. I also swam. Like Rockne, somehow I always managed to be on championship teams.

Sports was not the only school program I took advantage of before college.

Our music programs in school were also an instrumental part in teaching me and my mind-body coordination. I found this out in the marching band when we started creating formations during halftime on the football field. I would sweat at least ten pounds during an August football game in Florida, having to wear a wool marching band uniform. I'm surprised no one passed out from heat exhaustion back then.

Recently, I found several studies proving the importance of music in our lives, especially learning how to play an instrument or singing. The study found that folks who played an instrument or sang in a choir scored higher in math classes from all the years we learned how to count beats and measures in music.

The study also stated that folks who were in music programs were less likely to commit suicide because music helps release feelings and emotions.

I was watching an episode of the reality music show *American Idol*, on which Steven Tyler was a judge. Before his career as a judge on *American Idol*, Tyler was known as the lead singer of Aerosmith.

After one of the finalists performed a song he wrote, Steven welled up with tears, put his hand on his heart, and told the singer, "I could feel your heart."

He went on: "Art is an expression of our hearts. Perhaps we wouldn't choose to put horrible things in our bodies if we could express our hearts the way you just did."

It was a beautiful and gut-wrenching comment from a man who has struggled with substance abuse over a long and successful career as a rock star.

I learned more about my health as I got older.

Entering college was overwhelming. I was addicted to Diet Coke. The sodium from the Diet Coke was being absorbed by my body, preventing my halo to stay above my head. By this point, it was falling to my waistline. I was sixty pounds overweight.

I had been known to get off work, eat a whole pumpkin pie, and wash it down with a six-pack of Diet Coke or Tab.

I was only concerned with my physical body, denying any responsibility other than blaming hormones and the stress of college life.

I was taking a full load of classes at college and holding down two jobs to pay for my books and tuition.

My mother and sister Tammy would now become my life/body coaches. Tammy struggled through high school with her weight. During college, she was faced with the same health challenge as I was. Neither of us was morbidly obese; we were headed that way if we didn't get a handle on it, and we knew the health risk involved.

It was time to take charge and create my own wellness program.

I can hear my mother's voice to this day whispering to me, "You didn't gain it overnight; you're not going to lose it overnight."

We talked about creating an exercise and diet program. After listening to my mom's and Tammy's coaching about food and what to eat, I would always sit in silence and ponder our conversations to see what was applicable and what was not.

I advise you do this when creating your wellness program. If anyone or anything does not resonate with what you are feeling, it will not work. You are the one who has to commit to yourself. No one else. You have to stay disciplined and dedicated to your process.

Again I can hear Mom say, "According to the Bible, it takes twenty-one days to create or form a new habit and only three days to break it."

Great, I thought. Twice as long and hard to get my body back into shape.

After looking at myself in the mirror, I realized I had to take responsibility for the choices I had made to get me here, sixty pounds overweight at the age of twenty-five. I weighed 194 pounds and was a size 16, after years of always being 134 pounds and a size 8. Yikes! Now I was starting to feel depressed.

After making a commitment to myself to eat better and to be healthier, I solicited the help of my mom and Tammy to keep me in line.

Tammy came up with the one-handed or finger rule. This was similar to the rule we used when learning how to read except instead of using books, we would use food.

When choosing a book for class, the teacher would tell us to use one hand, pick up the book, start reading the first chapter. For every word we could not pronounce or understand the meaning, curl your finger up underneath the book cover. If you end up curling all four fingers, you'd drop the book, which meant it was too advanced, and you'd need to put that book aside until you chose another book to complete for your book report.

Tammy was reminding me of this method and applying it to what we eat.

When going to the food store, I was to pick up all packaged foods with one hand, look at the label, and read the ingredients listed. For every ingredient I could not pronounce or did not know, I was supposed to curl a finger. If I ended up curling all four fingers and dropping the packaged food, it wasn't healthy for me. It is a simple rule I still use today.

Mom and Tammy also started coaching me on diets created by other people. Mom was old-school. She believed in a proper square meal, reducing caloric intake, and exercising.

Tammy took it a step further and applied it to the Fit America diet, using food combining as well as exercising for good results.

Following any diet usually means cooking in more and eating out less.

This was the diet I would embrace for the next twenty-five years, until my sister Tammy turned me on to *The Bulletproof Diet*, by David Asprey, which talks more about the food-combination theory than Fit America and addresses the fast pace of life.

Asprey acknowledges that we live in a stressful world. Most people worry that they can look and feel better, but they are not because of their food choices. He researched foods that give us more energy than others.

After adjusting my diet, I realized a lot of my social activities were centered around eating.

Now I had to convince my friends to exercise activities. This ended up being easier than I thought. We all joined the gym, started walking or biking. We would also go "tubing" down the Ichetucknee River in Florida, a clear, spring-fed stream, which meant swimming as well. Nothing like seventy-two-degree water to get your heart going. In the Florida heat, it felt glorious as we swam and frolicked and moved our bodies in the sun.

Although my life became enriched with outdoor activities, it was not enough to melt the sixty pounds away. However, I got off to a good start with fifteen pounds.

It was time to look at other alternatives. So I read Jim Fixx's *The Complete Book of Running*. Fixx inspired me, like he did many other Americans, to join the fitness revolution by jogging. However, when he died of a heart attack while running, I had to reevaluate my workout plan.

So one day, sitting outside the gym, my friend Susan, who is a dancer for the local ballet, suggested I start walking instead.

Susan asked me which I would rather have, a lean sleek body like a dancer or a short stocky body like a lot of soccer players we knew.

I quickly answered a lean sleek body, of course. She then encouraged me to walk, claiming walking lengthened the muscles in our legs, where running shortened them, giving us a bulkier look.

I then thought of Frank Shorter, the long-distance marathon runner who trained for the Olympics in Gainesville. He won a gold medal in the 1972 Olympics. When I asked her about him, Susan reminded me of his body type. Of course, his body type was different than mine. Although I am tall for a woman, I have big bones and can bulk up very easily without even trying. Genetics, of course, plays into this too.

So I started walking four miles a day instead of running. I also changed my diet. Eating organic foods and less dairy as well as decreasing my sugar and wheat products. My diet now has a lot of monounsaturated fats, like avocados.

In my own research, I also learned that injury and inflammation in our blood vessels are often caused by the low-fat diet recommended for years by mainstream medicine.

Dwight Lundell, a heart surgeon in Arizona, says that the biggest culprits of chronic inflammation are quite simply the overloading of simple, highly processed carbohydrates (sugar, flour, and all the products made from them) and the excess consumption of omega-6 vegetable oils like soybean, corn, and sunflower, which are found in many processed foods.

Lundell claimed that the long-established dietary recommendations of a low-fat diet have created epidemics of obesity and diabetes, the consequences of which dwarf any historical plague in terms of mortality, human suffering, and dire economic consequences.

I lost the sixty pounds I had packed on within a few years after I discovered it was really my armor protecting my heart.

What else do I know? Well, during college I minored in children's literature and physical education. I met Dr. Hal Lerch, a physical education professor, who became my biggest inspiration for creating a fitness program close to home. Lerch said the closer your workout is to your front door, the fewer excuses you can come up with not to do it.

If a close-to-home approach is still challenging your lazy streak, start putting on your clothes. This always works for me, Lerch said.

The more I learned about Dr. Lerch and his own health story, the more I found myself feeling guilty for not taking better care of my body.

Lerch was a survivor of a skydiving accident years before when his parachute failed to open. Needless to say, he broke many bones and was temporarily unable to walk. He promised himself that when he learned how to walk again, he would run. He has been running in the Boston Marathon for over twenty years.

I had the privilege of covering him on his tenth anniversary Boston Marathon run in the eighties as a feature story for the *Gainesville Sun*, where I was a photojournalist for several years.

Today, reducing stress and living in a rural area with a lake, I can walk around with my dog, surrounded by wetlands and estates with thousands of acreage. This is now part of my maintenance program. I have gloriously clean air to breathe as I quickly take my 2.5-mile daily jaunt.

I continue to garden as much as I can, growing vegetables that I enjoy eating, knowing what fertilizers have not been put on them. I can also be around like-minded people.

Please do not make an excuse for yourself that you do not have an outdoor space for growing vegetables or that you cannot afford organic foods. There are plenty of indoor vegetable-garden kits that are compact and space friendly.

Another helpful key to the success of my exercise regimen includes my dog.

My furry family has taught me how important it is to honor animals in my life. Animals have been reported to reduce blood pressure and to keep us company.

At my house are Beau, a parti-colored English cocker spaniel; Henry, the Holstein cat, because his coat is patterned like a Holstein cow; May Day, the black beauty Bombay kitty who looks like a miniature panther; and the heavenly crew of cats Toby, Savannah, Winslow, and Timmy—all healers and coaches in their own right. I always knew when I had a healthy catch ready to cook because these little angels would often try to sneak a taste of salmon or shrimp before I could throw it on the grill. Timmy was known to make a nosedive in lots of shrimp salads, especially when out-of-town guest were visiting and leading the dinnertime prayer. As soon as our guests would bow their heads, he was taking a bow across the table with a piece of fish in tow.

Today, I carry Beau up and down thirty-one steps and push him in his dog jeep that looks like a baby stroller. We make a 2.2-mile loop around Hunns Lake almost every day. I do this as a reminder of how he and my cats have carried me and my heart so many times.

When it is snowing outside, I fantasize about sleeping in, but my sweet dog, Beau, reminds me that he still has to get up to take care of his needs. You know, the basic bodily functions and exercise that, if not taken care of promptly, make for extra-unpleasant chores to clean up afterward. This knowledge forces me to follow suit in accompanying him on those long walks. I think they help us both, and that is a good thing.

So, there you have it. My secrets to my body's fitness and well-being program that helps to keep me out of the hospital. I tell friends and family members that my wish for my body is to stay healthy enough and make enough money so I can die in my own house surrounded by love—something so funny that people laugh when they hear how.

What I have learned on my journey is this: our bodies are amazing. If you can keep your will in check, your body will take over.

It is really mind over matter or shall I say mind over chatter.

Chatter from our inner voices preventing us from making healthier choices to live heartier lives.

Chapter 13

You Are Responsible for You

Our mind means everything to our health. The ability to think and to reason is perhaps the most powerful function of our bodies.

I can remember growing up hearing my mom chanting, "A mind is a terrible thing to waste" while my brother and sister would watch television. Although as a family we would occasionally watch a television program or movie with our parents, Mom preferred that we read books to engage our minds.

She thought there were too many negative things that Hollywood television shows were exposing us to—off-color fiction—and she believed that they were distracting us from our higher source.

Mom kept watching about what we were consuming. Among our peers at school and television viewings, she quickly learned to limit our activity with both.

We did not go to church like some other family members or neighbors. However, I would watch my mom read the Bible and other books on spirituality—books like *I'm OK—You're OK*, by Thomas Anthony Harris, and others about positivity and spirituality. She claimed these books exercised her mind and kept it from being distracted from things that did not matter, allowing her to stay positive and to choose love.

Mom truly believed our minds created our reality. She also thought it was true that our minds, if not carefully used and disciplined, could lead us astray and separate us from things we wanted or the love we desired.

Books were my mom's salvation—and later in life, mine too.

Integrating the knowledge she gained from each one by practicing what she learned was crucial for her well-being and inner peace.

I called Mom's teachings the dance between our minds, ego, emotions, and spirit. I later learned from Mom and her books that the only way to live a healthy, happy life was to allow our minds to accept God as the leader of our dance—not our ego, emotions, or perceptions.

Harris's book *I'm OK—You're OK* was based on theories of transactional analysis. Transactional analysis is a system of popular psychology based on the idea that one's behavior and social relationships reflect an interchange between parental (critical and nurturing), adult (rational), and childlike (intuitive and dependent) aspects of personality established early in life by Eric Berne in 1958.

Berne wrote about his theory in greater detail in his book called *Games People Play*. Berne was convinced his theory was the blueprint of the mind, which no one had constructed before, along with a precise vocabulary allowing anybody the understanding to identify parts of the blueprint. This vocabulary made it possible for two or more people to talk about behavior and know what it meant.

Harris took Berne's work and summarized the three ego states: parent, adult, and child into "I'm OK—you're OK." They were outlined as "parent" (taught concepts), "child" (felt concepts), and the "adult" (learned concepts).

Harris had a long career in the navy as a psychiatrist,

leaving the military in 1954. Two years later, after starting a private practice in 1956, he became interested in collaborating with Bernes on the transactional-analysis theory.

Harris's book *I'm OK—You're OK* goes on to say that most people live out their lives in a negative—the "I'm not OK—you're OK" state—causing dysfunctional emotional reactions toward people around them. Harris's goal in his book was to inspire the reader to adopt the ideal "I'm OK—You're OK" mind-set.

Harris believed this attitude of "being ok with yourself and others" is the pathway to happiness, personal satisfaction, and healthy relationships. The phrase "I'm OK—you're OK" became an instant part of the American vocabulary.

Perhaps Louise Hay took Harris's theory a step further by looking at mental patterns learned by our minds that would later show up in our bodies in a dis-ease state.

Hay, in her book *You Can Heal Your Life*, goes on to share her hypothesis through her practice and her own life experiences.

Hay had been diagnosed with cancer. She had elected not to have surgery but to eradicate it by working from the inside out of her body by addressing her mental patterns. Hay had worked with enough clients to know that mental healing could work.

In 1978, thirty-nine years ago, life threw her a curveball or chance to prove to herself whether her theory would work. She was diagnosed with incurable cervical cancer. She believed the word *incurable* was not only frightening to many people but also meant to her the disease could not be healed by any outer means. So for her, the only choice was to go within.

Hay was raped when she was only five years old. She had

also been battered as a child. Hay, who died at age ninety on August 30, 2017, shared that there was no wonder why she manifested cancer in her cervix. She also understood cancer was a dis-ease of deep resentment that had been held for a long time until it literally ate away at her body.

Through her own self-discovery and examination, she realized she had refused to be willing to dissolve all the anger and resentment she carried at "them" over her childhood.

After a thorough mental and physical cleansing without surgery, six months after her diagnosis, Hay received a clean bill of health from her doctors. She was completely cancer-free. Hay can honestly say from her own personal experience that "*disease* can be healed, if we are willing to change the way we think and believe."

Hay's *You Can Heal Your Life* is a reference guide that I continue to use when I find something going on in my body—meaning a physical problem. I am always fascinated by chapter 15, "The List": "I am healthy, whole and complete." This is the list Hay created from her experience while working with clients in her practice. "The List" can be used as a guide to correlate dis-eases that you may have had or are having now and probable causes.

Hay recommends four things for us all to do in this chapter. First is to look up the mental cause associated with the area of the body or body parts where you are experiencing dis-ease and see if this could be true for you. If not, she encourages us to sit quietly and ask ourselves, "What could be the thoughts from our minds or in us that create this dis-ease?" Secondly, she wants us to repeat to ourselves, "I am willing to release the pattern in my consciousness that has created this condition." Thirdly, she suggests that we repeat the new thought pattern several more times. Finally, she says we should believe we are already in the process of healing.

Hay wrote at least ten other books to empower her readers to live happy and healthy lives. She ran her publishing company, called Hay House, as well as a charitable organization, called the Hay Foundation.

Although *You Can Heal Your Life* sits on my desk and is used periodically, Marianne Williamson's book *Return to Love: A Reflection on the Course in Miracles* is in heavy rotation. The daily lessons from the course and her lectures have influenced me the most in my life. They have helped me discipline my mind and strengthened my attitudinal muscles the most.

ACIM resonates with me because it is based on love—not fear. It also teaches us that our answers are within, not outside, of ourselves. This idea may feel foreign to a lot of cultures because it does not encourage seeking outside of ourselves for answers.

ACIM also talks about how our minds can create separation from one another and the love we desire.

How many of us have family members or friends who want to give us advice? This can be dangerous because what is true for them may not be true for you or me. Williamson believes in prayer and meditation and connecting with God, allowing him to provide each of us our own answers.

ACIM dissects the mind into five levels: desire, belief, thought, emotion, and perception.

One of the greatest blessings bestowed on me for living near New York City is Williamson's weekly lecture on ACIM, held at Manhattan's Marble Collegiate Church on Twenty-Ninth Street at Fifth Avenue each Tuesday night. This is the church our president, Donald Trump, attended as a little boy. My fellow ACIM students and I have created a wonderful like-minded community where we can grow and flourish.

Williamson's lecture has been worth the price of high New York taxes. Her gift is being able to take complex experiences in her own life, along with the wisdom of lessons she's learned, to share her knowledge—inspiring us all to live a simpler, happier, and healthier life through love and forgiveness.

A Course in Miracles was a book scribed by Helen Schucman and edited by Schucman and William Thetford, both professors of medical psychology at Columbia University's College of Physicians and Surgeons in New York City. It was written from 1965 to 1972. Schucman believed that the "inner dictation" came from Jesus.

The book is divided into three sections entitled "Text," "Workbook" (with 365 lessons), and a "Manual for Teachers."

According to Williamson, *A Course in Miracles* is a book about forgiveness—the psychological training in relinquishing a thought system based on fear and accepting, instead, a thought system based on love.

The thought system based on fear dominates our world. If you think about that notion, I think you can see that it's true. Williamson describes it as a mental filter through which we are taught to interpret things. Interpreting life through the mental filter of fear leads us to further thoughts of fear.

These thoughts of fear ultimately lead to feelings based on fear. Those will lead us toward behavior that is an expression of fear. The outcome of this fear-follow-fear thinking—a life that does not work.

That last phrase certainly rang true for me about a life that did not work.

And I interpret that line of thinking this way: when we live an ego-centered or driven life, there is never enough. The way you may recognize this in your own life is by being able to manifest on a material plane everything you thought would make you happy, like a lucrative job, a luxury car, a multimillion-dollar home in an affluent area, a vacation or weekend home in addition to your main house, fancy brand-name clothes, being able to travel for leisure any place in the world, or perhaps being married or in a partnership with an influential person in the community, but yet you feel something is missing. You are still not completely happy.

The fact is, all those external things cannot make you happy.

To our ego all these things spell success. Well, if this is true, why do you still feel empty inside while surrounded by the external prized possessions, the kind that most people would chop off their right arm for or want to trade places simply to have your lifestyle?

Our ego is very clever. It can also masquerade by showing up through cultural pressures from family and friends. The ego would view what you have manifested on the physical plane as a success.

I know this one to be true. I know this because this was my life four years ago. I had many material things, and yet I knew deep down that even with the trappings of the world that I had amassed, I was missing something far more substantive.

My friends and family members would give me their views and opinions about my romantic relationship, most of which were not true to what I was feeling. Or they would try to meddle. All this did was create more confusion, slow down my clarity, and frustrate me more. I loved them, but their best intentions were not a part of my private solutions.

When my best friend or a new friend who knew me only for a short while would ask how I was and if I was happy, after feeling my emptiness, I would quickly answer with a padded "fine." I knew he or she could feel that I was not wanting to address the real answer to his or her question. I also knew he or she was asking because he or she wanted me to know I was not alone and wanted to feel close to me because he or she loved me.

However, before I knew it, my ego would jump in and dismiss or devalue their motives. I could hear my ego justifying to myself that a new friend could not possibly know if I was happy or not. How could he or she possibly know me or my truth when he or she had not been in my life very long?

On a deeper level, the part of me that was craving love knew that my new friends cared enough about me to share their observations. I do know that there is a small percentage of people who are very in tune and intuitive. They do not have to know my story to know if I'm happy. They can feel if I'm happy or not by the energy they are feeling from me. This took bravery on their part to share what they saw and to ask.

Whereas most of my friends who were distracted in life by their own nonsense, who were in their own denial, were more invested in me liking them. Some would politely smile and tell me what I wanted to hear in case I rejected the truth. Those old friends were enabling me not to live in the light of love. It is the old crab-trap theory. When a crab tries to climb out of the trap, on its way out, the other crabs quickly grab it, holding it back so that the others do not have to do the work to be free.

Sometimes freedom may seem like we have to walk alone, but we are never alone. God is always with us—if we only allow him in. We connect to him through prayer and meditation.

ACIM has two basic categories that express themselves as we fall into this category of fearful thought and behavior: attack and defense. A primary cornerstone thought within the ego-thought system is the belief that someone is guilty.

The ego mind, or the loveless mind within us, is like a

scavenger dog, ACIM tells us. The ego is always on the lookout for any shred of evidence that our brother is guilty.

"Even when you take a stand and you are willing to extend your perception beyond your brother's guilt to the innocence that is the spiritual essence of who they are...the ego mind will often respond with you're right. They didn't do it, you did, you're the guilty one," Williamson said. "That is just as blasphemous as attacking anyone else. Because it is not only that your brother is essentially innocent in terms of who they really are, but so are you."

This vision of forgiveness that ACIM presents is different than the traditional notion of forgiveness. The traditional notion of forgiveness involves the belief that the guilt is real.

If you think that the world that we see with our physical eyes, that we hear with our ears and we touch with our hands, is ultimate reality, then people's guilt is real.

We all know people make mistakes. You make mistakes. I make mistakes.

Some mistakes are not that big of a deal. Although there are times in our lives that we make a huge deal about something that someone did, most of us can later look at that moment and with wisdom and see that it was not really that big of a deal at all.

However, some things that people do are a big deal—quite a big deal indeed—at least in moral terms.

Either way, ACIM would tell us that the realm of the physical body is three-dimensional. What we see. What we hear. What we touch. And it is not the ultimate real world.

It is described as real in ACIM with a small *r*. Beyond that, there is reality with a big *R*, and that reality with a big *R* is the only ultimate reality. The ultimate reality, she teaches, is the mind of God.

In her lecture on forgiveness, Williamson describes the mind of God as an infinite ocean of love.

"Now, in this world we are trained from the time that we are very, very, young to see the world and to think about the world according to the ego's fear-based dictates," Williamson says. "So from the time we're very, very young, unnatural fear-based thinking always caught within this polarity of attack-defense—attack-defense actually feels natural to us."

"What is actually natural thinking, which is the extension of love to all living things all the time, actually feels unnatural," Williamson says.

"So the salvation of the world is the salvation or deliverance from the mind-set that then produces all the horrors of the world," she says. "The mind-set being the ego-mind or fear-based thought system."

Forgiveness means that when we are standing in front of a loveless expression—somebody said something to you that you did not like or somebody was unkind to you or took something from you—when this happens we have to recognize that the entire world of somebody's behavior is the realm of the circumstance.

This is the realm of the physical body, but we can extend our perception beyond what the physical senses perceive to what the heart knows to be true.

"My eyes saw that nasty look on your face. My ears heard that sarcastic tone of voice. My hands can practically touch this...I know what's going on here," Williamson describes.

Forgiveness, according to ACIM, is my recognition that the real you is not expressing yourself at the moment when you are engaging in this uncomfortable behavior.

Because God created all of us as one, and we are all an idea in his mind, God is all that there is; therefore, what is all-encompassing can have no opposite, and anything that is happening in our three dimensions that is not an expression of love. This entire three-dimensional plane is itself an ultimate illusion.

The idea is that beyond this world, ACIM says, there is a world I want. But the world we want is not a world that is registered with your physical senses.

So forgiveness is where we extend our perception into the world we really want by knowing that it is there.

God's creation is all that is real.

ACIM sums it up:

"Nothing real can be threatened. Nothing unreal exists. Herein lies the peace of God."

To some, this depth of thinking about our behavior and the God inside us is outside the scope of understanding. What I have learned, however, is that ACIM is my EZPass to happiness.

It has become another way to measure if I am truly living my best life. If I am allowing God to flow through me during the day, I try to notice how the energy feels during activities. When accomplishing my daily tasks, does the energy feel free and flowing or forced?

If the energy feels free and flowing, this is God working through me. If it feels forced, this is probably ego driven or my own will, not God's.

I invite you to check out ACIM.

If you do not live in the New York City area, you can live-stream Williamson's lectures on ACIM weekly.

Williamson also has recorded each ACIM lesson, which you can order from her website. I ordered her downloads to be delivered to my email on a daily basis. Each day before I make human contact with the outside world, I download my ACIM lesson, meditate, and pray. It's my way to clear my mind and to invite God into my life to direct my day so I can get out of my own way.

The prayers I use to begin my day are simple ones.

I use the St. Francis prayer that my Grandma Connella taught me and Williamson's prayer "Where Would You Have Me Go?"

St. Francis:

Dear God, make me an instrument of Your peace. Where there is hatred, let me sow love; where there is injury, pardon; where there is doubt, faith; where there is despair, hope; where there is darkness, light; where there is sadness, joy.

O, Divine Master, grant that I may not so much seek to be consoled as to console; to be understood as to understand; to be loved as to love; For it is in giving that we receive; it is in pardoning that we are pardoned; it is in dying that we are born again to eternal life.

Marianne's prayer to God "Where Would You Have Me Go?" "Where would You have me go? What would You have me do? What would You have me say, and to whom?"

Our minds are like our bodies. They need constant exercise, devotion, and discipline to stay healthy. A clear mind is an answer to a peaceful life and healthy body. Forgiveness is the key to love.

I will close this chapter with a poem that I love, that brings me peace, from Rumi:

Let yourself be silently drawn by the stronger pull of what you really love.

The wound is the place where the Light enters you.

Don't grieve. Anything you lose comes round in another form.

Your task is not to seek for love, but merely to seek and find all the barriers within yourself that you have built against it.

Let the beauty we love be what we do.

Beyond ideas of wrong-doing and right-doing, there is a field. I'll meet you there. When the soul lies down in that grass the world is too full to talk about.

Lovers don't finally meet somewhere. They're in each other all along.

When you do things from your soul, you feel a river moving in you, a joy.

Why do you stay in prison when the door is so wide open?

If you are irritated by every rub, how will your mirror be polished?

Chapter 14

The Power of Our Spirit

During my mom's illness, after she was diagnosed, we would talk about spiritual things.

Mom would tell me just as our bodies have many parts, so does our spirit and our soul. Conscience, fellowship, and intuition are its three components.

Our conscience is for us to have the ability to discern right from wrong or to condemn. Mom would strongly advise me to listen to my conscience, especially to always live life and to tell the truth. I'd hear her say, "Let your conscience be your guide." She would warn me, if I didn't listen to my conscience, it would be easier and easier to drift into the shadow side of life.

Fellowship is for us to contact, connect, and commune with God as well as each other. Her motto was to see the God in each other and to do as God would want you to do, especially when no one was looking.

Lastly, intuition is a direct sense or feeling in our spirit regardless of the reasoning or circumstances. This is how our spirit perceives. If we're too busy or distracted, it's sometimes hard to listen to our intuition, especially when emotions are high or we're under pressure.

Our mind, emotion, and will are part of our soul. The mind is for thinking, considering, knowing, and remembering. In our minds, we have thoughts, ideas, concepts, reasonings, understanding, knowledge, and intelligence.

Our emotions are feelings, positive or negative, that make it possible to love or not.

Our will is the part of our soul through which we have purpose and choice to make decisions.

Mom would show me the Psalms, the book of the Bible that talked about these parts as "the hidden parts."

Our hearts are composed of our spirit, soul, and body.

God is the holy spirit within us all. In ACIM, it states that we are all God's children. No one is more special than the other.

Meditation and prayer are the way to communicate with God.

Mom taught me that when we do this, our lives become more meaningful. She would ask me to watch and listen to people in my life.

God puts people in our lives for a reason, she'd tell me. God's spirit works through you and me to connect our spirit with the spirits of other living beings. Our spirit may not know the exact story in the moment, but on a deeper level, we can feel a connection to someone else's spirit or even an animal's spirit. These connections could be for an instant or a lifetime.

Our spiritual connections can be a blessing as well as a healing to our hearts.

Mom would also tell me that not everyone could or would be my friend. You can count your true friends on one hand. True friends will experience all of life with us without ever giving up on us.

"A blacksmith does his best work when the fire is the hottest," she would say when she felt like I had a fair weathered friend around. It's easy to love someone when life is fun. But when the chips are down and work is ahead, a true friend will stand beside you and start working with you to get through the tough time.

Mom and I would call these friends Ts, T standing for a true friend. A true friend was someone who could go deep on the vertical plane, which is the base or vertical line of the T, but yet enjoyed life on the surface. Life on the surface is the cap of the T, or horizontal plane or the horizontal line. Going deep all the time would be too intense but having fun keeps us alive when appropriate. I say appropriate because to think life should always be fun is not healthy or real.

One true friend came into my life unexpectedly. Our journey began on Thursday afternoon in August 2016, when around 1:00 p.m. I received a page on my work cell phone for an NPWT device order. The name on the order was one that I vaguely recognized. The last name took me back to when I covered Stamford, Connecticut, for our high-risk-obstetric company.

I remembered one obstetrics resident from the early 2000s. We first met when she covered labor and delivery at Stamford Hospital. I would have to go there with our high-risk-pregnancy company's nurse, May-Helen, to meet with Dr. Viscarello as we helped to get his patients started on our service before they were discharged.

Several hours later, around 4:00 p.m., my work cell pinged to tell me I had a new email in my work account. I looked at it quickly because I was trying to get off from work so I could pick up my niece, Amanda, from JFK Airport. Amanda was set to visit me for the first time on her own without her parents. I had planned to take Friday off to show Amanda around and to create memorable aunt-niece experiences and deepen our connection.

The email was from our customer service department forwarding an email from the physician assistant who had ordered NPWT for the patient I got a page from earlier. He needed help and wanted to set up an appointment that Friday because it had been a long time since he had a patient on NPWT.

By now it was almost 6:00 p.m., and Amanda's plane was supposed to land around 8:30 p.m. It took me about an hour and a half or so to get to JFK, and I wanted to be on time to give Amanda a warm welcome. JFK can be overwhelming for travelers who have never experienced one of the biggest multicultural airports in the world.

But duty to our patients called. I took a deep breath and called the cell phone number the PA had sent me. While dialing, I saw the town Yonkers come up on my screen underneath his phone number.

My mind started to wonder, and I thought if he lived in Yonkers, I could meet him along my route off of I-87, the New York Thruway, to JFK Airport and give him a brief refresher demonstration.

The PA, named Al, answered. He was so grateful and kind that I actually answered his email so quickly. He explained to me that his patient was an ob-gyn who was one of the most generous and kind people he knew. He further explained that the wife of the physician who owned the practice he worked for had done her residency with this patient, who was also a physician.

Once he shared that this patient was an ob-gyn I knew, I had to open my heart even wider. I have a soft spot because I watch so many ob-gyns give up parts of their lives to serve their patients. I saw throughout my career in obstetrics, female ob-gyns who were parents themselves would miss out on some of their own kids' events to be on call. Al kept telling me how much this physician cared so much about her patients and how he wanted to extend her the same courtesy.

While talking to Al, I was reminded of Cheri Hubert's book *The Key: And the Name of the Key Is Willingness.* This book is yet another book based on ACIM. In her book, Hubert suggests that only by willingness can we recognize that in the material world, what we give away we no longer have and that in the spiritual world, only what we give away do we have.

As you can imagine, I started to struggle on a deeper level with myself, which was not normal for me in a situation like this. For some reason, my inner voice kept calling me back to this patient. I thought it was very interesting because normally I don't struggle with my inner voice. But because it was coming from a deeper place, I knew I had no choice but to honor what I was feeling. I knew I was being guided by a higher source, God.

I was being called on to join the circle of love among healthcare professionals. Giving our gift by putting *care* in healthcare. This is exactly why I was attracted to working in healthcare from the start. Healthcare allows me to show my heart to others through my role as a medical-device representative. It sounded like Al and this patient felt the same way. They were, it seemed, my kindred spirits.

So I told Al that the timing was not great—I was off when he wanted me to be there with him to help his patient with her NPWT device. But as we discussed this, I learned that although Al was nowhere near Yonkers, he lived about thirty-five miles south of me, off of I-684. This route was even better because that was on my original route to the airport.

I rushed to move things from my work car to my personal vehicle, taking the NPWT equipment with me. I also loaded in my dog, Beau, who typically travels with me because of his age. We agreed to meet off of exit 6. In addition, I emailed Al some explanatory videos on how the NPWT device is used. I thought this would give him more confidence for his appointment the next morning so that even though I could not get there to help, he would feel empowered to handle it.

I was curious about his patient too.

As I pulled into the parking lot where Al had instructed me to go, I saw this handsome man waving me into a spot next to where he was parked. Keep in mind, Al and I were both meeting well after office hours were over for this patient. I did not know him, and he did not know me. I climbed out of my car. Al rushed over to introduce himself as I pressed the button inside my car to lift the back hatch, exposing my roadside classroom. He then patted me on the back and welcomed me.

We both looked at each other, our faces lighting up with a huge smile of gratitude, and thanked each other for meeting. He knew I was in a hurry to get to the airport for my niece, and I knew he had his son's football game to attend.

As my roadside class ended, I made sure Al had my work cell phone number and told him I would be available by phone if he had any questions.

I know, you're thinking I am such a sucker, right? Again, I kept feeling this deeper connection, and I had not even spoken to his patient yet.

The next day arrived, and now I had Amanda with me. It was Friday afternoon, and I found myself wondering how Al had done with our patient. While Amanda was busy checking in with family at home, I called Al to see how things had gone.

Before I knew it, he invited me to join him in his office on Tuesday afternoon for the first dressing change. I graciously accepted.

On Tuesday, I entered the lobby of AMI Surgery, the office where he worked. I noticed the profile of a stunning, short, dark-haired Persian woman sitting on the couch. Her purse, about the size of my roller bag luggage, was tucked behind her legs. She was covered in lots of swanky baubles and was scrolling through her texts while talking on her phone.

Within in a few minutes, I spotted her NPWT device in its pouch hanging off her left shoulder. After she hung up from her telephone conversation, I gracefully walked over and introduced myself. I then asked her about her experience of being on the NPWT device and about her wound.

As she looked up, our eyes met. I felt her energy, and my heart quickened. It felt authentic. We both stopped all chatter and gazed deeply into each other's eyes. We were silent for a few moments, and then we both let out smiles that lit up each other's faces.

It was a smile of recognition and an instant camaraderie.

Shieva, as I found out her name, then shared with me that she had been diagnosed with ovarian cancer. Unfortunately, her laparoscopic hysterectomy and staging for her ovarian cancer were complicated by a bladder perforation that had necessitated a low vertical incision to repair it.

Her physician quickly followed her surgery up with chemotherapy, which caused a major delay in her wound healing. In fact, even worse, it ultimately created a very large wound opening that needed an NPWT device to close.

After she explained how she pronounces her name, Shieva Ghofrany, she began telling me about her experience and her diagnosis, and I suddenly remembered why her name sounded familiar. Just as I suspected, I had met her when I worked with Dr. Viscarello years before at Stamford Hospital. Shieva was the chief resident.

I shared with her that when I had seen the page come up on my phone with her name, I had this instant feeling of knowing.

Most people might not have known what I meant by that statement—a feeling of knowing. She did. Shieva verbalized her reciprocal feeling of connectedness when meeting me.

I handed her my business card. Before I could close my briefcase, she asked me about my name because Shary Connella was highlighted with my title and position. My work email address as printed was mary.connella@*******.com.

Shieva was already trying to figure my story out and seemed just as intrigued with me as I was with her. I could feel us both simultaneously feeling the energy between us. Then Al stepped in and interrupted us to do her dressing change.

Shieva was hilarious. Despite her condition, she had a wicked wit. She was charming, engaging, and didn't miss a trick. Her mind was always a step ahead of us.

Before Al could remove her dressing, she would be handing it to him. She was quick, precise, and didn't like to pussyfoot around. She wanted to get in and get out so she could get back to her patients.

At forty-six, she was a partner in a large ob-gyn practice in Stamford, Connecticut. She was also married to a man who could give George Clooney a run for his money. They have three kids. She was the breadwinner of her family, so she had to continue working while she received treatment for cancer.

My head was spinning and my heart broke all at once when she shared her circumstances. A sick physician having to care for others. There would be for her even when she needed it the most.

This weighed heavily on me—she was so young, and so were her kids. And I think her story hit home even more for me when I found out she had ovarian cancer. Although I am careful not to project my situation onto her, I could not help but think of when I had my myoma. I was 46 too. I believe this was God showing me a replay in of way so I could help this woman.

Although our situations were different in a lot of ways, they were also similar. I knew what it was to have a lot of people depend on me. I also was strong, independent, and a fast study.

Al had to leave the room for a few minutes. Shieva started asking me questions about my life. As we swapped stories, I looked into her eyes. She looked back, and without saying anything else, I felt the connection deepen between us.

We finished her dressing change, and as I was about to bid her farewell, she asked me if I could come back for all her dressing changes. Although I had never done this for any other patient, I wanted to grant her wish.

The office manager and Shieva, who lived locally, announced they would like to start doing her dressing changes as early as possible. This meant 8:00 a.m. for them and 5:00 a.m. for me because I lived an hour and a half away. You have to understand, I have no problem getting up when needed for work, but 5:00 a.m. is not my best hour.

Despite the early hour, for two months, twice a week, I'd meet Shieva for her dressing change. I began to look forward to our early-morning meetings. Shieva fascinated me with her knowledge of Eastern medicine. Most traditional physicians are trained in Western medicine, and very few are open to stepping outside those boundaries, especially when treating cancer with chemotherapy.

I then learned that Shieva had audited a two-year graduate program in integrated health and healing at the Graduate

Institute in Bethany, Connecticut, which is helmed by Bernie Siegel, MD, its academic codirector.

It was at integrated health and healing where she learned the harmonious functioning of all the dimensions in treating her patients. The dimensions include corporeal, energetic, emotional, mental, interpersonal, consciential, and spiritual.

This approach embraces biological, chemical, medical, and surgical tools and psychological, sociological, cultural, spiritual, and environmental ones, which traditional medicine doesn't do. I studied a lot about this at massage school as well as on my own with my own health challenges.

Before, during, and after her office visits, we would discuss books, practitioners, cultures, foods, philosophies. I would leave with eagerness to get home and find a new book as if it were the next adventure to take Shieva on.

We'd turn each other on to books the other hadn't read.

Finally, I had found a spiritual playmate who used all modalities to heal the body. This had been rare for me to find. I relished in our quest and hunger to learn more. I loved Shieva's curiosity.

We also illuminated each other's hearts in a way that hadn't been felt in a long time.

After Shieva was discharged from our services, she would text me pictures of her most prized and treasured possessions: her kids. I would follow by sending pictures of my furry family since I had never had children. I'd also send her pictures of my home. She really wanted to come to visit my home, especially since I had been to her home. She was tired from her chemotherapy treatment, and I didn't want her to feel pressured or obligated.

Her home was an extension of her, filled with so many meaningful touches celebrating her life and family.

The uncanniest thing about my connection with Shieva was I had made a pact with myself not to allow anyone else into my heart again in any way. I had just come out of a seventeen-year relationship with an ob-gyn and was pretty shut down to any invitation, much less a close friendship.

Shieva called it "no longer accepting any new members to my friendship club." But there was something about her that melted away all my defenses and opened my heart. When she told me her last name Ghofrany meant "forgiveness," I had to shake my head because her friendship made me forget about my broken heart. It was as if she helped me heal my invisible wounds, and I helped her heal her surgical wound.

We were helping each other create scars.

As such, I would find myself continuing to include Shieva and her family in my daily prayers. After praying for her body to be healed free of cancer and any other disease, I prayed for her happiness.

Have you ever prayed for someone's happiness? Try it right now. When you say "happiness" out loud in a soft voice, hear the emphasis on the *ss*. It's almost as if you're whispering "shhh"—sending an invisible hug to that person and giving yourself one right back as you offer up your happiness prayer to them.

In a letter Shieva wrote to my boss after my asking her to share her experience of working with me, she noted, "Having cancer is, in many ways, a terrible ordeal as one can imagine, though as I have said many times since my diagnosis on June 17, 2016—many silver linings were offered up to me," she said. "not the least of which was meeting Shary Connella!"

Shieva continued, "Shary really shows that the 'people' behind the device (often more important than the device itself!) are an integral part of the process."

Perhaps God's spirit orchestrated Shieva and I meeting again to heal our body, mind, and spirit as well as our hearts. I call this being in the divine flow. Mom would definitely call Shieva a T.

You'll know when you are experiencing the divine flow with someone because it feels so loving and magical all at once—almost like rising in love instead of falling.

I often smile when I reminisce about meeting Shieva again, almost twenty years later. What a beautiful reminder that we are all connected to each other and to God through our spirits. We just have to make a connection with him every day through meditation and prayer.

Love is not formed from the physical body. Love is formed through our spiritual connection. And love, I believe, is our most powerful tool for health and also healing.

Chapter 15

It Does *Take a Village*

In 1998, shortly after Mom's diagnosis, our family was blown away by our community's generosity.

As word got out that she was very ill, well wishes for a speedy recovery poured in. Flowers, food, cards, plants, even housekeepers—any way someone could express his or her love or support for our mother showed up to offer solidarity in our time of despair.

Our communities are the fabric of our lives. We all need community. When I use the word *community*, I mean it can be more than one community. For me, it can be family, friends, or fellow ACIM students, healthcare professionals, photographers, animal lovers, neighbors, church or Facebook buddies, the world. For you, it could mean other platforms or groups.

Community represents parts of our lives that feed our souls and spirits on a deeper level. We share common interests or bonds.

When I returned to New York for work in January 1999, after being with Mom, I will always remember what Dr. Nancy Kirshenbaum had me do.

I had been rounding on labor and delivery (L&D). I had only met Dr. Nancy Kirshenbaum a couple of times since starting with the high-risk obstetrics company four months prior. She was a maternal-fetal medicine specialist, also known as a perinatologist, a high-risk ob-gyn at Westchester Medical Center and my number one prescriber in New York.

Dr. Kirshenbaum asked me if it was true what her nurses had shared—that my mom was terminally sick with a rare disease. I sadly shook my head up and down and replied, "Unfortunately yes."

She then took out her script pad and wrote an address on it and asked me to give her a ten-minute start before I left and to meet her as soon as I could get there. Not knowing where this was or what this was about, I agreed.

The address turned out to be her home. She introduced me to her husband and three kids as well as her housekeeper and said to me, "Our home is your home. You are always welcome here." She then went on to share that when she was away at medical school, her mother had been diagnosed with a very aggressive form of ovarian cancer. She only got to come home once to see her mom before she passed.

Nancy knew what it was like to be so far away while having her mother so sick. She wanted me to feel loved and a part of her family.

I teared up in appreciation for her gratitude and generosity. Nancy and her family became my beacon of light. She would continue to throw me a lifeline on the days that she could read that I must have gotten unfavorable news from home in Florida.

Nancy's friendship was invaluable. And what she did for me—extend herself in my time of crisis—was very rare.

You see, today we are living in a culture of separation—from ourselves and our fellow humans. Most of us live separated from nature as well. Contrast this with the interconnected way of life that is still practiced in a few places on our planet today.

In these communities, a person lives as part of his or her community—the tribe—and the tribe, in turn, lives as an integral part of the surrounding nature. I'm not suggesting we should return to such tribal cultures, but we can develop similar but contemporary forms of community that reflect our cultural history and moral compass—dedicated to the outreach of one another's hearts.

In this way, we make a conscious decision to live in a community—and one that includes a diversity of people complementing and supporting one another in their growth. By growth, I mean to not only see and shape our own beings but to take on the responsibility that goes beyond ourselves. This ability to understand and know ourselves, within the human context of a group and the ecological context of planet Earth, grows when we live in a community that supports our spiritual connections and does so without trying to change a person's individuality or desires.

"Let us think of ways to motivate one another to acts of love and good works. And let us not neglect our meeting together, as some people do, but encourage one another" (Heb. 10:24-25, New Living Translation [NLT]).

My uncle Bootsie (a.k.a. Clarence Edward Connella), our dad's youngest brother, who is a retired fire chief in Alexandria, Louisiana, echoes Scott Peck's belief. Peck said in his book *A Road Less Traveled*, "There can be no vulnerability without risk; there can be no community without vulnerability; there can be no peace, and ultimately no life, without community."

Uncle Bootsie says man was not created to live alone. We need one another. And what I love most about living in New York is that most New Yorkers live by Uncle Bootsie's credence, especially in the New York Police Department, New York Fire

Department, and our healthcare communities. When one of our own falls, we gather in record speed to rally, to lift up our fallen colleague. We also lift his or her family up.

Our community can create miracles when we work together.

On September 11, 2001, perhaps our nation's greatest tragedy unfolded, but a silver lining was exposed as we watched how our magnificent NYPD, NYFD, healthcare teams, and volunteers from across the United States and around the world came out in force to aid New York City in a time of crisis. People who didn't have to come responded without hesitation. With determination. With pride. And our nation felt connected.

It was amid this era that I had the opportunity to meet Marianne Williamson for the first time. Williamson was a spiritual leader of the 2,300-member Renaissance Unity Church in Warren, Michigan at the time. She offered her own help to our community in prayer and out of love.

Looking back, I think most communities are very much like ours in New York. We're actually all one community throughout the world.

On a Saturday in June 2017, Beau and I took off at 4:30 a.m. on a two-day driving trip from our home in Stanfordville, New York, to Alachua, Florida. Alachua is a small town just outside Gainesville, home to the University of Florida. It's a long time behind the wheel.

The last few hours of this ambitious driving trip, I had fantasies about sleeping in until at least 9:00 a.m. the next day. But no such luck. My dad is an early riser, and so is my sister Tammy. I could hear them talking downstairs as if they were both in bed with me. However, when I turned to look at the pillows next to me in bed, no one was there. Dad and Tammy's voices carried the tune of my alarm clock.

Tammy and her husband, Dale, drove down from Charlotte, North Carolina, my sister Melody and her husband, Chris, flew in from San Jose, California, and my brother, Tommy, and his wife, Rhonda, were driving up from Tampa, Florida.

All of my siblings and I were home in Gainesville to celebrate with our hometown community a memorial tribute service for our friend Carla Hotvedt Pomar's life. She had just earned her wings to heaven after a long battle with B-cell lymphoma. Carla was our chosen sister, meaning that although she was not related by blood, our family loved her as if she were.

Carla had helped our family so much in our life; it was our turn to be there for her. Like it or not, our family went full throttle to help her as she battled a difficult disease.

It started with our uncle Sidney, who had been diagnosed before Carla with B-cell lymphoma. He had insisted she allow him and our family to help her. She would end up having the same specialist that both he and our mother had at Stanford Healthcare in Palo Alto, California.

Once back at her home in Gainesville, Carla would end up under the care of my mom's oncologist, Dr. James Lynch.

I met Carla while working at the *Gainesville Sun* newspaper during my college years. She was one of our full-time staff photographers. She was also one of the most prolific photojournalism teachers I have ever had. Carla and her husband, Julio, and I were also housemates for a time.

Carla was kind, intuitive, and empathetic. She was known to many for her photo story about Michael Hammond ("the Crisco Kid") in 1980. Although this little boy had a horrific skin disease, Carla had allowed her compassion, sensitivity, and the sweetness of that little boy to guide her through this assignment. Her impactful images had left his legacy with our community while giving us all a deeper understanding or feeling of what it must have been like to be this little boy.

Her images belied her giant heart.

Carla was also responsible for my break into photojournalism. She had recommended to her staff of photographers that they allow me to shoot a photo assignment so they could celebrate one of the intern's birthdays.

I will never forget her confidence in me. Sometimes, I think she believed more in me as a photojournalist than I did. She reminded me of my talents during her class, encouraging me to feel like I could do this assignment with ease. She also stood ready to help, reminding me that she was just a phone call away, and if I needed her to assist in developing my film, she would.

Keep in mind that these were the days before digital photography and pagination. We still photographed assignments with film. After we would shoot an assignment, we would rush back to the darkroom to develop and print before the copydesk deadline.

Our cameras did not have a screen on the back like they do now. Images did not magically and automatically appear within fractions of a second after pushing the camera release button. Photographers had to rely on their skills, learning about lighting before leaving our subjects. There was no margin of error allowed. We didn't have Photoshop to pull a rabbit out of a hat in case our flash didn't fire correctly.

After returning to the *Gainesville Sun* darkroom and before I could get my roll of film out of my camera, I heard the phone ring. It was Carla. She wanted to see how things went. I was excited, of course. My first photojournalism shoot for our newspaper. I quickly answered that it was so much fun! Thanks for recommending me, I told her, and then asked how her party was going.

Carla laughed because she knew I was on a deadline, and we really did not have time to chitchat. "Do you need my help to roll the film onto the reel?" she asked. Rolling film onto a steel reel is tricky until you get the hang of it. If you are not good at it, you can damage your entire roll of film and thus muck up your assignment.

Although I thought it was kind and supportive of her to want to come into the office to help me be successful with my first assignment, I wanted her to enjoy herself. I graciously thanked her, and with confidence answered, "I think I've got it."

The next morning, guess who showed up at my front door with a copy of the newspaper containing my first published assignment? Carla. She wanted to be the first one to congratulate me.

That was Carla. Supportive of everyone's talents. And so it was not surprising that most of our *Gainesville Sun* colleagues from the eighties gathered alongside our families and friends to celebrate all that Carla had meant to us. Some flew from far away, making time in busy schedules to honor her considerable role in their lives.

I was not expecting to see Dr. Lynch at this gathering. Dr. Lynch had taken care of Carla for sixteen years or so. But there he was, stepping up to speak, sharing with us all what Carla had taught him as his patient.

Dr. Lynch started out by saying the word, "Remembrances."

"Human knowledge is never contained in one person. It grows from the relationships we create between each other and the world, and still it is never complete," he spoke.

"There is a moment, a cusp when the sum of gathered experience is worn down by the details of living. We are never so wise as when we live in this moment," he said.

"Science may provide the most useful way to organize

empirical, reproducible, data, but its power to do so is predicated on its inability to grasp the most central aspects of human life: hope, fear, love, hate, beauty, envy, honor, weakness, striving, suffering, virtue."

He continued: "The physician's duty is not to stave off death or return patients to their old lives but to take into our arms a patient and family whose lives have disintegrated and work until they can stand back up and face, and make sense of, their own existence."

"Those burdens are what make medicine holy and wholly impossible: in taking up another's cross, one must sometimes get crushed by the weight," he shared.

"I am blessed with the most wonderful patients, and I continue to learn more about how to live with truth and grace blended. She was a patient for sure, but more than that a friend, a sister, and a wonderful encouragement to me. I have her picture watching over me daily as I work."

We then heard him end his wise and emotional tribute with scripture, a verse from Ecclesiastes: "It is better to go to a house of mourning than to go to a house of feasting, for death is the destiny of everyone; the living should take this to heart."

After Dr. Lynch concluded, I got to speak with him about Mom and Carla. We then started sharing our experiences and thoughts about healthcare in America. We both agreed on two things. The first was, we are in serious times. Our healthcare system is in a crisis. The second was that we agreed on a fix. The only medical remedy for our healthcare system is a single-payer system, like Medicare for all.

Back to our sense of community.

If a picture is worth a thousand words, then I think a thousand thoughts are worth an action. We need one another, every man, woman, and child, to come together as one community to pressure our politicians to give us a single-payer healthcare system in America. We are the only country out of the six wealthiest in the world not to have a single-payer system. Canada, the United Kingdom, Finland, Australia, and Iceland's citizens do not have to worry they will lose their life savings to a healthcare crisis like many Americans face every day of their life.

I wonder if these six countries have lower cancer rates than Americans because of less worry. These six countries are proof we can have a single-payer system. These six countries look at America as the leader in wealth, but yet our own country's healthcare system is about to crash. Why not embrace this healthcare system model and show the rest of the world how to do it the best?

Uncle Sam and Aunt Shary *need you now*! We can do this together, and I think it is time for all of us to be spurred to action. Let's march like our ancestors before. Had the Reverend Martin Luther King Jr. not marched in 1963, seeking civil rights for women and blacks, today blacks might not have the right to vote. Such bold but peaceful activism was surely powerful.

The Voting Rights Act was signed into law by President Lyndon Johnson on August 6, 1965, eliminating legal barriers at the state and local levels that had prevented African Americans from exercising their right to vote under the Fifteenth Amendment to the Constitution.

It is our community as one nation that encourages our actions to come from the heart. It is unthinkable that our politicians would all have Cadillac healthcare policies but not the people who elected them. Does not this imbalance sound as ridiculous, nearly, as the history around black voting rights? One group of people should not benefit above others when it comes to matters of health.

America was not built on this inhuman ideology—that some of its citizens enjoy rights that another class, culture, or race do not. It was built on liberty—for all. And that includes access to quality healthcare—perhaps our new frontier in civil rights.

Liberty comes from the love of mankind. Love comes from above, and I believe it moves inside our hearts when we join as one for the good of all.

Let's strengthen our communities and overturn this toxic healthcare system together—and create a healthier national program for all Americans.

Chapter 16

Our Time Is Now

In August 2017, Kaiser Health News reported the results of a new public opinion survey that found that American physicians are warming up to a single-payer system. I was not surprised by the findings.

Although I find this interesting that Kaiser Health News would report this since it was Edgar Kaiser who was responsible for the beginning of our healthcare crisis.

In 1973, Nixon did a personal favor for his friend and campaign financier Edgar Kaiser, then president and chairman of Kaiser Permanente. Nixon signed into law the Health Maintenance Organization Act of 1973, in which medical insurance agencies, hospitals, clinics and even doctors could begin functioning as for-profit business entities instead of the service organizations they were intended to be.

I know that when I spoke to Dr. Lynch, the oncologist who attended my mother and my friend Carla, he explained that he had privately supported such an idea for years. He and I agreed on a single-payer system because as healthcare

It's no longer enough to have a high-paying salary, a great insurance policy, and significant life savings. People who are diagnosed with terminal illnesses or cancers are losing their jobs, insurance policies, money, homes, and for some, even their marriages. Because one major illness just takes them down in one ferocious life-altering tumble.

Wouldn't it be awesome if our healthcare professionals didn't have to deal with the red tape and paperwork they encounter each day? You know what I mean. The kind of red tape that leads to frustrating delays in making your appointment. And often, the kinds of delays that compromise the quality of care you get during your checkup or physical exam.

You have a problem. You know it is getting worse. And they can see you to check it out—two months later. We have all been there. And it is frustrating, if not scary, especially when our medical issues are concerning.

We have also seen the pages of insurance paperwork we must fill out, as required by physicians, so that we can have a test or procedure done.

We have also heard stories about folks who agree to healthcare coverage on one date and paid for their contracts, only to find out that the procedure they specifically needed is no longer covered. The insurer simply shifted gears and posted its latest changes in coverage on its website without you knowing.

We are all at the mercy of their shenanigans. And for many of us, that often life-and-death shell game is wearing thin.

For that reason, we're now seeing new public opinion surveys showing that the majority of Americans now support a single-payer system. Many who have been on the fence have now fully had it with the red tape. They want simplicity, certainty, and quality care.

If Canada, Australia, the United Kingdom, Finland, and Iceland, all developed countries, have been successful in using a single-payer system, why can't America? I believe we can do it more cost-effectively and for less than what each of us is now paying with our healthcare premiums and taxes—and in a way that would be fairer.

I am not immune to the blowback. Critics of single-payer have argued that it is tantamount to socialized medicine. But if we really consider where we are, we already have socialized medicine. It's called Medicare and Medicaid. The reason why it is not working for us is because we've complicated our healthcare system with corporate America. By allowing big business through private insurance companies to dominate our healthcare market in America, we have allowed them to get rich at the cost of people's lives.

We must flip-flop our healthcare coverage model in America so that Medicare for all will become the dominating force. And then, private insurance companies can supplement the rest.

Outspoken billionaire Mark Cuban has argued that folks who have addictive personalities will still have health issues. OK. I agree with him. However, under my single-payer system, those who are addicted to food, cigarettes, and alcohol would be paying for their own healthcare, whereas presently they are not. You and I, as tax-paying citizens, are further enabling them by not requiring them to be part of the solution.

I know from my own experience, if I invest in something, whether it is time or money, I am more engaged in a positive outcome.

Think about my two-cent national sales tax plan. Even if we have to raise this percentage a little, it would be less than what we are currently paying and with more transparency—which is a good thing.

Everyone who is in our country, regardless if they are a resident or a visitor, would contribute to our healthcare system. God forbid something to happen to a tourist while vacationing in America, but if something did, they too would be covered by the taxes they pay during their journey.

I also think my suggested system would reduce fraud because our healthcare fund would be coming from one source, not several, which would make it easier to trace or to follow the money trail.

An added bonus. Our overburdened physicians could then do what they do best: examine, diagnose, and treat patients, focused not on government overreach but on providing quality healthcare.

One model I like, and one we should consider, is that of Denmark.

U.S. News & World Report, in a recent magazine survey, ranked Denmark's healthcare system number one on the planet—*not America,* but tiny Denmark. It's a universal public healthcare system that is funded largely by taxes and administered by local municipalities.

Denmark's residents receive primary care from general practitioners through services run by private physicians who contract with the municipalities. The physicians there are paid on a mixed per capita and fee-for-service basis. Most hospitals are also run by municipalities. Only about 1 percent of hospital beds are in the private sector.

There is another bonus. Denmark also happens to be ranked as the world's happiest country. And in some respects, I would imagine many citizens there are happy because they can rest easy at night not having to worry if they will lose their jobs, their homes, or their mates if they become sick.

I will also note that the Danish diets and lifestyles are also healthier than those in the United States. I believe that is another key to improving our American healthcare system. We need to refocus on being responsible for healthier choices—what we are putting in or around our bodies as well as keeping them in motion with exercise. The burden of good healthcare cannot solely rest in a system. It must also support personal responsibility. All of us can do just a little bit better by making even small changes in that regard. It's a small step forward, but one that pays big dividends for us all.

I believe we should do everything humanly possible to stay out of the physician's office or the hospital. Do not get me wrong. If I were to get in a serious car accident or have an acute episode like a heart attack that required hospital assistance—get me there in a New York minute.

However, I truly believe we can avoid having to seek treatment if we have healthier, more loving relationships with our bodies, and that includes nurturing healthier minds and spirits. It all works together.

I know there are some Americans who do not believe socialized medicine could work in America, but that is not true. These are the same folks who are enjoying Medicare or Medicaid, which is a form of socialized medicine signed by President Lyndon Johnson in 1965. We just do not connect the dots that the formulas are the same.

Every American who is employed or self-employed funds these two programs by paying federal income taxes, state taxes, payroll taxes, and FICA (the Federal Insurance Contributions Act)—a tax made up by Social Security and Medicare taxes.

According to a study by the Tax Foundation, the average American worker paid a 31.5 percent tax—a figure that combines 15.7 percent income tax and a 15.9 percent payroll tax. The average worker in this study earned an annual income of $50,084.

In 2017, the Medicare tax rate was 1.45 percent on the first $200,000 of earnings. Keep in mind, this is not including your property tax rate—a tax that some owners may pay for patients who live in their area and are hospitalized and receiving care. Our property taxes help pay this off too.

If you are self-employed, the maximum 15.3 percent self-employment tax rate is on your first $127,000 of self-employment income, which is up $8,700 from 2016. If your income is above $127,200, an additional 2.9 percent Medicare tax is charged to you.

Medicaid is funded from three primary sources: 41 percent of general revenues, 38 percent from payroll taxes, and 13 percent from beneficiary premiums. Medicare Part A is financed by 2.9 percent tax on earnings paid by our employers and you the employee, which only account for 87 percent of Part A revenue.

See what I mean about our complicated system? Perhaps this is why our country's healthcare system is failing. If our government makes it so complicated for us to follow, we cannot hold them accountable or see that we pay twice as much if not more than countries who have a single-payer system.

For all of these reasons, I am deeply concerned. We are America—the land of the free—the most prosperous place on earth. And even with all of our fabulous determination, we continue to have a healthcare crisis in this country.

Hospitals are closing. People and their families who once held prestigious jobs with high-paying salaries and great insurance are falling short. All it takes is one illness or injury to ruin their responsible planning in life and wipe out their hard work and success. It could be any one of us who has been frugal, who has saved, who has worked multiple jobs and raised strong families. The system could take us down and destroy our lives.

We can no longer bury our heads in the sand. We have to

take to the streets like our ancestors before us. I believe it has come that far, that it has gotten that bad.

Perhaps people like Bernie Sanders, from our political sphere, or Marianne Williamson, from our spiritual cadre, will soon become our generation's leaders on this issue. Like Mahatma Gandhi and the Reverend Dr. Martin Luther King Jr., who led their own movements, we need to engage in nonviolent protests to bring attention to our healthcare problem. If we gathered millions throughout the country to march in solidarity, it would send a strong signal to our politicians that we deserve the same insurance they have.

Americans can no longer tolerate or accept our politicians' ways of thinking when it comes to our healthcare system. This gridlock has been nearly single-handedly created by political discord and power mongering—to allow our politicians to have a lifetime of premium healthcare without providing us the same is ludicrous.

Let's review our Declaration of Independence.

It begins:

> *In congress, July 4, 1776, the unanimous Declaration of the thirteen united States of America,*
>
> *When in the Course of human events, it becomes necessary for one people to dissolve the political bands which have connected them with another, and to assume among the powers of the earth, the separate and equal station to which the Laws of Nature and of Nature's God entitle them, a decent respect to the opinions of mankind requires that they should declare the causes which impel them to the separation.*
>
> *We hold these truths to be self-evident, that all men are created equal, that they are endowed by their*

Creator with certain unalienable Rights, that among these are Life, Liberty and the pursuit of Happiness.

That to secure these rights, Governments are instituted among Men, deriving their just powers from the consent of the governed, That whenever any Form of Government becomes destructive of these ends, it is the Right of the People to alter or to abolish it, and to institute new Government, laying its foundation on such principles and organizing its powers in such form, as to them shall seem most likely to effect their Safety and Happiness.

So our time is now!

"We the People of the United States" need to stand up for each other. We need to join together as one nation and demand a single-payer system.

As it states in the Constitution of the United States:"We the People of the United States, in Order to form a more perfect Union, establish Justice, insure domestic Tranquility, provide for the common defense, promote the general welfare, and secure the Blessings of Liberty to ourselves and our Posterity, do ordain and establish this Constitution for the United States of America."

Isn't losing your job, your home, your spouse, and your savings threatening your security and your happiness as stated in the Constitution? I believe it is. I truly do.

Isn't our current healthcare crisis challenging our general welfare instead of promoting it? Isn't our current healthcare system threatening our security? It seems to me, at least on a broader level, that our current system violates our Constitution.

And after studying this document, I have concluded that

our politicians giving themselves the right to a lifetime of the best health insurance, and not including you and me, is a breach of the Constitution—upon which our country was built.

It is true that our country has created and made many advances in technology and treatment. But whose life would be worth living if you had to lose everything in order to live? Especially after working hard all your life to take care of yourself—and then, after you have become seriously ill, finding out that you make too much money to qualify for financial assistance that might prevent you from losing your home, your savings, and your marriage.

Let me be clear. It is not brotherly love—or love for your fellow American or love for your country—to allow Americans to live under a healthcare system that can jeopardize our well-being as humans on this earth.

We have a serious healthcare crisis, and it will take you and me to fix it—not Washington, where stagnation has led to zero progress on the healthcare front.

We need a total shift in perception to create the miracle that will change our nation's healthcare systems. Healthcare should *not* be trusted as a business—not a commodity, a trade, a product, or a car service.

Healthcare also cannot be run like the typical Wall Street business model, where two plus two equals four. That is why our current healthcare system is failing. And I think that it is crushing to look back and realize that healthcare in the sixties and early seventies, before HMOs became popular, ran better than it does today.

We have become over transactional—looking at nearly everything as to how it can benefit us personally—not all of us but a few. I believe we are off course in following this path.

If I go back to the time of my birth, when Kennedy was in our White House, neighbors cared about one another. This is how my parents raised me. We need to return to that way of thinking again.

We should use our own moral compass—rely not on our politicians but on one another. The difference between when I grew up and now is that we did the right thing for our country—not the popular thing but the right thing. And for all of us.

This is not a time for neutrality. That is a silent position, and silence means agreement. Again, I argue that we deserve the same healthcare benefits that our lawmakers have given themselves. To do less for the rest of us is un-American.

I have observed in my own decades of work—seen firsthand—that it is not your doctor or any other healthcare professional delaying your care. It is the current system we are in. Healthcare professionals went into healthcare to make a difference in our community and to help take care of patients so they would live longer, fuller, healthier lives. And the system has now taken away much of their control to do so.

We have to look underneath the surface of our healthcare crisis to fix it—to look deeper in order to stop this bleeding of our well-being and livelihoods.

The system does not make it easy for you to understand. Try to read every page of the Affordable Care Act. It's insanely detailed and long, loaded with the same kind of bureaucratic base covering that makes people, even many lawmakers, shake their heads.

Some might argue that the people who wrote it counted on you not reading it. I'm not that cynical, but I do believe that it is incumbent on you as a consumer to do your research rather than rely on media to tell you what you need to know. In many cases, the folks sharing the news are telling you exactly what the big business of healthcare wants them to—and these talking heads, who have zero expertise in healthcare, don't know the difference.

Start doing your own homework. Do not rely on only one news source; instead, listen to all sides and separate the political bickering and power mongering from the truth. Look at who funds campaigns and who carries favor from the healthcare industry with lawmakers. Review the chapter in this book on healthcare executive salaries and compensation. Call your local senator, and tell him or her that you demand a single-payer system or at least the same healthcare coverage he or she has for the same cost.

If other countries can have a single-payer system for healthcare, America can too! Other countries look at America to be the leader. And I think we can be, making our new system run better than any other country in the world! How do I know this? 'Cause we are America, the greatest country on earth, and we are Americans—a name that ends in *can*.

I return to the story my mother and her brother, my uncle Sidney, read to me when I was young called "The Little Engine That Could," by Watty Piper.

"I think I can, I think I can, I think I can..." the little engine said.

And *we can too*!

Let's put the heart back into America's healthcare. Put healthcare—put it first over profiteering.

In hospitals, the phrase *code: blue* signals an all-hands-on-deck emergency, a frantic call for doctors and nurses to stop what they are doing and save someone.

I am calling for a code: red, white, and blue—for our country.

Our current healthcare system is dying. Let us band together to not only make it thrive but also to keep it alive for our children and generations ahead.

Without your health, you have nothing!

Acknowledgments

I would like to express my eternal gratitude to the many people who saw me through this book—to all those who provided support, talked things over, read, wrote, offered comments, allowed me to quote their remarks, and assisted in the editing, contributing, and proofreading.

I would also like to thank my team of proofreaders and contributors: Andrea Billups, Pam Louis, May-Helen Hildreth, Stephen Hayes Kattell, Alexandra Harris, Kristen Kunkle-Somma, Stelli Munnis, Donald McGrath, Kristin Lombardi, Jodi Stone Goachee, Elaina Garcia, Deborah Tribero Temple, David Albert Temple, Daisy Joplin, and Susan and Peter Lehmann. Above all, I want to thank my sister Tammy and my furry family (Beau, Henry, and May Day), as well as the rest of my family and friends who supported and encouraged me along the way.

Lastly, I would like to thank Joe Carr, of Joe Carr Photography, for creating the original *Code: Red, White, and Blue* button.